Ignite Your Holistic Journey

Discovering Nature's Secrets and Unlocking the Holistic Edge

D. R. Darcy

Table of Contents

TABLE OF CONTENTS 1

INTRODUCTION 4

CHAPTER 1: UNVEILING RADIANCE: HOLISTIC CARE FOR YOUR HEAD
AND HAIR 6

WHAT IS HAIR AND HOW DOES IT ACTUALLY GROW? 7
Hair Follicles 7
Hair Growth 8
FOUNDATIONS OF HEALTHY HAIR 10
The Scalp 11
Hair Types 12
WHOLE-BODY NUTRITION FOR HEALTHY HAIR 15
ANCIENT HEALING INGREDIENTS FOR TOPICAL HAIR CARE 17
Recipe: Lavender Stress-Relief Scalp Massage Oil 19
Recipe: Rosemary and Aloe Vera Hair Mask 20

CHAPTER 2: GLOWING COMPLEXION: UNLEASHING THE HOLISTIC
POWER OF YOUR FACE AND SKIN 22

SIMPLE PRACTICES FOR RADIANT SKIN 24
RADIANT NUTRITION: EATING FOR HEALTHY SKIN 27
Skin-Friendly Foods 29
TOPICAL SKIN CARE 31
Nature's Pharmacy: Plant-Based Skincare Ingredients 31
Recipe: Green Tea and Witch Hazel Facial Toner 34
Recipe: Turmeric Face Mask 35

CHAPTER 3: SERENITY UNLEASHED: HARMONIZING YOUR NECK AND
SHOULDERS THROUGH HOLISTIC PRACTICES 38

UNDERSTANDING NECK AND SHOULDER TENSION 39
HOLISTIC TECHNIQUES FOR UPPER BACK BODY TENSION RELIEF 42
HARNESSING THE POWER OF NATURE: NATURAL INGREDIENTS FOR GENTLE BACK
CARE 45
Remedy: Soothing Neck-and-Shoulder Herbal Compress 47

Remedy: Eucalyptus and Peppermint Balm 48

CHAPTER 4: HEART'S SYMPHONY: NURTURING HOLISTIC HARMONY IN YOUR CHEST AND HEART...50

HEART-HEALTHY NUTRITION: NOURISHING YOUR CARDIOVASCULAR SYSTEM 53
HEART-HEALTHY MOVEMENT 55
CULTIVATING EMOTIONAL WELLBEING: THE HEART-MIND CONNECTION 57
ANCIENT WISDOM: NATURAL INGREDIENTS FOR HEART HEALTH......................59
Recipe: Garlic and Hawthorn Tonic................................61
Recipe: Turmeric Golden Milk.......................................62

CHAPTER 5: DIGESTIVE VITALITY: UNLOCKING THE SYNERGY OF HOLISTIC WELLNESS IN YOUR DIGESTIVE SYSTEM 64

GO WITH YOUR GUT: SUPPORTING YOUR GUT MICROBIOME.........................66
THE MIND-GUT CONNECTION...69
HEALING HERBS AND SPICES FOR DIGESTIVE SUPPORT 71
Recipe: Gut-Soothing Ginger and Lemon Infusion 74
Recipe: Fennel and Papaya Salad 75

CHAPTER 6: FOUNDATION OF STRENGTH: REVITALIZING YOUR LEGS AND FEET WITH HOLISTIC SYNERGY 76

REST AND RECOVERY: HOLISTIC TECHNIQUES FOR TIRED LEGS AND FEET 78
Energizing Movement: Exercise for Lower Body Wellbeing...........81
SOOTHING REMEDIES FOR HAPPY FEET AND LEGS.................................83
Remedy: Potato Foot Mask for Aching Feet 84
Recipe: Turmeric and Ginger Foot Soak 85

CHAPTER 7: THE HOLISTIC NEXUS: CULTIVATING SYNERGISTIC WELLBEING FOR YOUR BODY, MIND, AND SPIRIT...........................86

BUILDING MEANING INTO DAILY LIFE..87
REDISCOVERING BALANCE: NURTURING THE BODY-MIND-SPIRIT CONNECTION ...89
Body-Based Practices for Enhancing Inner Harmony 92
Ingredients That Feed Your Soul 93
Recipe: Ashwagandha Elixir.......................................95

CHAPTER 8: INNER RADIANCE: UNLOCKING THE SYNERGY OF HOLISTIC HEALING FOR YOUR MIND...96

HOLISTIC APPROACHES TO CULTIVATING MENTAL WELLBEING 97
NUTRITION TO ENHANCE COGNITIVE FUNCTION..................................100

Recipe: Brain-Boosting Ginkgo Biloba Smoothie *103*

CHAPTER 9: INNER SYMPHONY: HOLISTIC SUPPORT FOR OPTIMAL ORGAN HARMONY AND BALANCE **104**

THE INTERNAL ORGANS 105
The Liver *106*
The Kidneys *106*
The Lungs *107*
The Pancreas *107*
STRENGTHENING VITAL ORGANS: A HOLISTIC APPROACH 108
HERBS AND FOODS FOR ORGAN HEALTH 110
SUPPORTING DETOXIFICATION AND CLEANSING 112
Recipe: Detoxifying Dandelion Tea *113*

CHAPTER 10: SYNERGISTIC NUTRITION: FUELING YOUR BODY AND MIND **114**

CREATING A BALANCED PLATE: THE WELL-ROUNDED APPROACH 115
Superfoods for Vitality and Wellness *119*
Harnessing the Power of Herbs and Spices: A Flavorful Path to Health *122*

CONCLUSION **126**

REFERENCES **128**

Introduction

Recently, a close friend called me to ask if I'd ever heard of sunscreen pills, and whether I would recommend those. Yes, you read that correctly: Pills that are meant to protect you against UV damage. Of course, I told him that these pills have been proven to be ineffective—as have various other health fads, such as crystal-encrusted water bottles, appetite-suppressing lollipops, oxygen shots, and numerous other treatments that offer promises of perfect health and beauty with the popping of a single pill. Since you're reading this, I'm guessing that you, too, are tired of the constant distractions and fragmented approaches to wellbeing that surround us from all sides. It can be hard to tell what's real and what isn't when every brand tries to market its new "wonder cure." This is why many of us feel a deep longing to return to simplicity, to natural ingredients, to use ancient knowledge to support our bodies and heal them from the inside. The truth is none of us need to drink a million different supplements, nor jump on the newest wonder cure bandwagon. All we need to do is use the wisdom of cultures that have practiced medicine long before brand-awareness and marketing was even a thing. Now, more than ever, it is essential to embrace the power of a holistic perspective.

The word "holistic" is derived from the Greek word "holos," meaning "whole." Holistic approaches focus on the whole person, rather than on a singular aspect; it represents a comprehensive approach that considers the whole person—in their body, mind, and spirit—in the pursuit of optimal wellbeing. It recognizes that we are interconnected beings, and that true wellness can only be achieved when we nurture and balance all aspects of our being.

In our quest for holistic wellness, we are not only exploring more recent evidence-based practices, but are also drawing upon the wisdom of traditional healing systems and the richness of cultural diversity. Our understanding of health and wellness is profoundly shaped by the diverse tapestry of human experiences, with each culture bringing its unique insights and practices to the table. Across human history, traditional healing practices, folk medicine, culinary traditions, and natural healing methods have been used and passed down from generation to generation, offering a treasure trove of knowledge and wisdom. These practices remind us of our innate connection to the natural world and the profound impact it can have on our wellbeing.

We will explore the remarkable potential of natural resources for whole body-health. From the medicinal properties of plants to the healing power of deep breathing, we will delve into a wide range of practices and techniques that can empower you to take charge of your own wellbeing. You will gain insights into the power of nutrition, movement, stress management, and spiritual practices to foster a harmonious and vibrant existence.

As we explore the vast terrains of holistic health, remember that this journey is unique to you. I encourage you to listen to your intuition, embrace your own cultural heritage, and adapt the practices and teachings to suit your respective individual needs. The path to holistic wellness is not a "one-size-fits-all approach," but a personalized and empowering experience that honors your body's wisdom. Open your heart and mind to the possibilities that lie ahead. Together, let us embrace the interconnectedness of our beings and with nature, and embark on a journey toward a vibrant wellbeing. Are you ready to embark on this transformative journey?

Chapter 1:

Unveiling Radiance: Holistic Care for Your Head and Hair

One of the most wonderful ways in which we, humans, declare our individual uniqueness is through our hair. Afros, bobs, dreadlocks, crew cuts, and pixie styles... There are almost as many hairstyles as there are people in the world, and wearing your hair exactly as you like can be an act of true creativity and liberation. On the other hand, hair care and styling can become quite a headache—sometimes, literally, when we try to pull and force our hair into shapes it doesn't naturally grow as.

Many of us sometimes feel at the mercy of our genes when it comes to the hair we have inherited; I've had many friends over the years complain to me about their thin, flat hair, which they wish was voluminous instead, or about their locks' tendency to frizz. It is true that our DNA plays a huge role in whether or not our hair is curly or straight, in its texture and thickness, and, of course, in your hair color. If you are of African descent, then your hair would tend to grow in a very different way than the hair of a Scandinavian person. The first step in holistic self-care is to understand and accept yourself as who and what you are, with your perceived limitations and genetic predispositions. It is from this place of self-acceptance that good self-care can really grow, since the energy you previously spent resisting your unique biology can now be spent on caring for your wonderful self. Seeming limitations are also doors into endless possibility, as we learn to play with, and love, the bodies we were born with. This definitely applies to hair care as well—as much as you might wish your hair were different, accepting your hair, and even becoming curious about it, is an important first step toward accessing health and radiance.

What is Hair and How Does it Actually Grow?

Hair is body tissue, just like skin, muscle, and bone. However, what makes hair so unique is that it is actually made of dead tissue; while your scalp is very much alive, and new hair sprouts from live cells, the long strands—called the hair shaft—that grow out are not technically "alive." They are made of keratin, a type of protein from which fingernails are also chiefly made. However, although the hair shaft isn't alive, it can still remain healthy or become damaged, as we'll see in the rest of this chapter. Furthermore, your hair is nourished by the blood vessels in your scalp, and thus good scalp care is very important to ensure that your hair grows well.

Hair Follicles

Each hair shaft grows out of a follicle, and every person is born with every hair follicle that they will ever have—about five million of them (Hollister, 2017). The hair follicle is really where the magic happens. It is a small, bulb-shaped gland that grows just beneath the skin, and it determines the shape and nature of each person's hair. If your hair follicles are round, then your hair will be straight, while oval-shaped follicles give rise to more curly hair. Interestingly, hair follicles can change shape throughout your life! Hormones, diet, and significant changes in lifestyle can often affect this. I have a family member whose hair, which had always been poker straight, grew back very curly after she had undergone chemotherapy. She had always wished for curly hair, and so this change was a very welcome side-effect of an otherwise invasive and unpleasant medical treatment. Perhaps you have experienced some changes in hair texture or color yourself, particularly when entering puberty or midlife, which is when many people's hair changes the most. It is also possible to consciously affect the shape and nature of your hair follicles, through making natural hormonal and dietary changes—within limits, of course. What is definitely possible is to ensure that your hair follicles are healthy, thus ensuring thick and luxuriant hair. In fact, that's what this whole chapter is about.

Hair follicles produce sebum, which is the natural oil that the human skin makes to protect us from the more damaging effects of the sun and air. As with the actual shape of the hair follicle, sebum production is affected by a host of different factors and can change many times over throughout our lives. As a teenager, for instance, you may have lamented the fact that your hair is very oily—meaning that you were producing a lot of sebum—while later in life, you may notice your hair becoming dry quite easily. Neither of these things is bad, and whichever stage of life you find yourself in, there are many strategies you can adopt to take optimal care of your hair.

Hair Growth

Hair grows in three stages: The first stage, which can last a few years, is called the "anagen phase." This is when hair grows enthusiastically. After that comes the "catagen stage," during which hair growth slows down and hair follicles start shrinking. The last stage, called "telogen," is when hair growth stops entirely and the hair eventually detaches from the follicle. After that, a new hair will emerge from the same follicle. At any given point in your life, you will have many hair shafts in every one of these three categories: About 90% will be in the anagen phase, thus growing vigorously, while some hair strands will be slowing down (thus entering the catagen stage), and other hair will be falling out, thus being in the telogen stage. Therefore, losing some hair every day is entirely normal, as long as you are not losing more hair than you are producing. Each hair follicle is capable of producing a new strand of hair about 20 times throughout your lifetime. If you consider the fact that hair can grow for several years before reaching the telogen stage and falling out, then you will quickly realize that some daily hair loss is hardly a cause for worry.

On an average, hair grows at a rate of half an inch per month, meaning that within seven years, if left to its own devices, hair can easily grow down to your waist. Interestingly, this applies to both men and women—in fact, the difference between women and men's hair is so minute that not even forensic tests can reliably distinguish between the two. The larger difference, of course, is that men more frequently go bald as they near middle age, but in terms of hair texture, there is hardly any difference.

Speaking of baldness—like other unique hair traits, such as having thin or thick hair, dark or blonde—there are some things you can do to delay or modify this trait, but in many cases, eventual balding is inevitable. Male pattern balding, in particular, is due to the presence of male sex hormones, called androgens, of which testosterone is the most important. Testosterone fulfills many important health functions, and so, although it is possible to suppress testosterone production in your body (which would slow the rate of balding), it is not advisable. However, there is some good news, since even with balding the hair follicles remain alive, which does mean that taking good care of your hair follicles could protect you from eventual baldness. We will discuss these strategies in later sections of this chapter.

Of course, the point of holistic health is that your entire being is affected by everything you do, and that nothing in your body happens in isolation. Good hair care also means taking good care of your gut, moving regularly, and cultivating practices that nourish both your body and soul. And so, as we move through this book and explore further aspects of holistic wellness, you will find strategies listed in other chapters that will also impact the health and vibrancy of your hair. For instance, when I began paying more attention to the quality of my sleep, my hair suddenly became healthier as well. My friend, Mary, began taking collagen supplements for bone density, and found to her surprise that her hair started growing thicker and more luxuriant than it had ever done before. And I've had many friends and acquaintances over the years who have discovered, to their surprise, that developing a gratitude practice, or simply learning to accept themselves as they are, has markedly improved the health of their skin, hair, and digestive systems. Learning to love ourselves exactly for who we are can, ironically, often change us more than any amount of sweat and effort possibly could.

Foundations of Healthy Hair

Now that we understand the basics of hair, I'd like to encourage you to spend a moment thinking about your own hair. Chances are you have done that many times in the past, often in the context of wishing your hair were different than how it is—more than any other body part, hair withstands an incredible amount of manhandling from us. We heat it, straighten it, curl it, color it, yet it continues growing. I'm not suggesting that you stop styling your hair however you want, but rather that you take a long, non-judgmental look at what you are working with. Self-knowledge will enable you to apply the best holistic and herbal treatments, tailored for your specific needs.

The Scalp

Let's begin with the scalp, the foundation for healthy hair. There are three main types of scalps—generally classified as oily, dry, and balanced—which are determined by how much sebum your scalp produces. Like other aspects of your hair, your scalp is subject to changes throughout your life, as your hormones fluctuate. Your hormones, in turn, affect the pH of your skin. Human skin tends to be on the acidic side, with the optimum pH of your scalp being 5.5. Hair itself is highly acidic—about 3.7—and for the hair shaft to seal successfully, it needs a scalp that is also slightly acidic. Many problems with our scalps such as dry, itchy scalp, or hair that is too oily—often caused by excess sebum production—is actually the result of a pH imbalance.

At this point, try to think about your own scalp, and about how it has tended to react to life events over the years. For instance, you may have found yourself in a seemingly endless cycle of washing your hair regularly, only to find that it becomes oily again within a day which gradually causes you to wash it more and more, yet with similar oily results. This often happens because shampoos strip our scalps of their natural oils and alkalize our scalps. In response, our bodies' natural regulators decide to produce more sebum, causing your hair to appear more oily, quite faster. If you do struggle with oily scalp and hair, then your body's natural tendency is to over-react to chemical products or hormonal fluctuations by acidifying your scalp in response. The best solution is to apply a 'less is more' approach, cutting down on chemical treatments and allowing your scalp to gently adjust its own pH as it becomes less irritated by outside influences.

On the other hand, if you find that your scalp is often dry and irritated, or that your hair itself is dry or frizzy, then you probably have alkaline hair and scalp. As I mentioned earlier, a high pH (which means alkalinity) prevents the hair shaft from sealing, leaving it more prone to becoming damaged and your scalp to becoming flaky. Interestingly, the first step you'll need to take, if that is the case, is the same as with an acidic scalp: Cut down on chemical products and treatments. Once your scalp becomes less irritated by external products, you can begin introducing gentle treatments that will not upset your own natural balance.

Hair Types

Unlike the scalp, which is as alive as the rest of your skin, the hair shaft itself is actually made of dead cells. This might sound strange, particularly because hair is often seen as one of the most vibrant aspects of our appearance. Yet, it is only the hair root that is actually alive, which is why scalp care becomes so vital. Although not technically alive, however, hair can still be damaged. The hair shaft needs to remain sealed to, for instance, prevent split ends and breakage. Frizzy hair is often the result of such damage, and is characterized by unruly, flyaway strands caused by moisture imbalances and open hair cuticles. To prevent this, regardless of your hair type, you should try to avoid using very strong bases (such as harsh soaps and detergents) on your hair which heighten the pH and cause damage. The first point of departure with hair care is to primarily focus on the scalp which determines the health of your hair shaft for the duration of its growth.

Different hair types have different needs, too, of course. Our hair is as unique as our fingerprints—varying in texture, thickness, and structure from one individual to another. Understanding your hair type is crucial for adopting a hair care routine that suits your specific needs and promotes healthy, luscious hair growth. While we now know that the scalp and hair follicles are the main determining factors of how your hair will appear, hair shaft type also plays a significant role in determining our hair's overall characteristics. The three primary hair shaft types are straight, wavy, and curly, which are, as we discussed earlier, determined by our follicles. However, within this, there is much variation. Two important variables are hair density—how many follicles you have, and how close your hair is spaced together on your head—and individual hair strand texture. You probably already know how dense your hair is, based on how voluminous it is. But do you know whether your individual hair strands are thick or thin? To figure that out, take a look at a few individual hair strands. Do they appear thick, almost like a guitar string, or is each hair strand almost invisibly thin? Neither is good nor bad, but this will have an effect on your hair care. Darker hair is also usually thicker in texture than blonde hair.

To summarize: Hair type can be defined according to four variables, namely color, follicle shape (whether or not your hair is curly), hair density (how much hair you have), and texture (how thick each hair is). It is entirely possible to have very fine, but abundant, brown hair, or curly, thick blonde hair, or wiry dark hair that is not very dense, or any combination of these. Caring for each hair type requires tailored approaches, but to begin with, here are some general tips:

- For straight hair, especially if the hair also has a fine texture, or if your scalp tends to be oily, avoiding heavy products that weigh down the hair is essential. Opt for lightweight conditioners and hair treatments to add body and bounce. Regular trims help maintain a polished look, as straight hair is more prone to showing split ends. When using home-made hair care products, focus on gentle moisturizing ingredients, or products that add protein, such as making a hair mask from raw egg (add some essential oils to mask the smell, although it will wash out easily and leave no lingering egg smell).

- If you have wavy hair, embracing your natural wave pattern is key. Don't overbrush your hair, since this will separate the hair strands and cause a frizzier look, and if possible, allow your hair to dry naturally. Use products that deeply moisturize your scalp without adding too much oil, such as yogurt and jojoba oil.

- Curly hair demands extra moisture to retain its shape and prevent dryness and frizz. Look for hydrating shampoos and conditioners, specifically designed for curly hair. If your hair texture is quite thick and wiry, then you can also use thicker oils such as coconut or almond oil, which allows the curls to form naturally without excessive manipulation.

- If your hair feels very heavy, either due to a coarse hair texture or simply because you have very dense hair growth, focus on providing regular moisture by using something like aloe gel or a light spray made of rose water and witch hazel. Also consider cutting your hair into a shorter style which can allow heavy hair the freedom to curl and grow in a more lighthearted manner.

- If your hair texture is quite fine, or your hair density itself is thin, then avoid heavy conditioners at the roots, as they can weigh down your hair and make it appear oily. Instead, focus on good scalp care, making sure your pH remains balanced, and cut your hair into a style that flatters the gentle fall of your hair.

- Regardless of hair type, protecting it from excessive heat and UV damage is crucial. Limit the use of heat-styling tools and avoid overly rigorous towel-drying as well. If your hair damages easily, then try washing it in lukewarm water rather than very hot water, and finish off with a cool water rinse to close the hair cuticles and add shine.

Whole-Body Nutrition for Healthy Hair

When it comes to achieving vibrant and healthy hair, proper nutrition plays a crucial role. The foods we eat supply the essential nutrients that promote hair growth, strength, and overall vitality. In addition to external hair care practices, incorporating a well-rounded, nutrient-rich diet can significantly impact the health and appearance of our hair. Hormones also play a key role in hair growth and health, while hormonal imbalances can contribute to hair loss, thinning, or slow growth. Maintaining hormonal balance is essential for optimal hair health, and certain natural supplements, minerals, and foods can support hormone regulation. Here are a few foods, minerals and herbs that support healthy hair:

- **Zinc:** This mineral helps regulate hormone levels, particularly androgen levels (which are responsible for male pattern balding), and supports the growth and repair of hair tissue. Foods rich in zinc include oysters, beef, pumpkin seeds, and spinach; adding a daily zinc supplement to your self-care routine could also be beneficial.

- **Vitamin B7 (also known as biotin):** Biotin supports the production of keratin, the protein that forms the structure of hair strands. Consuming foods high in biotin, such as eggs, almonds, sweet potatoes, and avocados, will strengthen your hair and help it grow more abundantly.

- **Omega-3 fatty acids:** Found in fatty fish like salmon, sardines, and mackerel, as well as in flaxseed oil, these fatty acids are very beneficial for hair health as well as skin wellbeing. These healthy fats provide nourishment to the hair follicles and scalp, promoting strong and lustrous hair. Additionally, omega-3 fatty acids have anti-inflammatory properties that can help combat certain scalp conditions that may hinder hair growth.

- **Vitamin E:** This is a potent antioxidant that supports healthy hair growth by promoting blood circulation to the scalp. Foods rich in vitamin E include sunflower seeds, almonds, spinach, and avocados. You can also buy vitamin E oil, and apply it directly to your hair as a deep conditioner or hair mask.

- **Saw palmetto:** This is a popular herbal supplement which is known for its potential to inhibit the conversion of testosterone to dihydrotestosterone (DHT), which is associated with hair loss. Consider using this as a regular supplement if you are suffering from hair loss.

Because the human body is such a sensitive and interconnected system, it is also important to ensure that your gut and other internal organs are healthy, too. If you find that your hair is very limp, or that your scalp is excessively oily or flaky, then it may be the right time to focus on your gut health in particular, as well as your endocrine system and blood circulation. Later chapters will cover how to take care of these systems in greater detail.

Ancient Healing Ingredients for Topical Hair Care

Having looked at the different hair types and their varying needs, and having addressed the need for whole-body nutrition, let's now take a look at some of the most widely used and beneficial hair care ingredients. Carrier oils are oils such as almond oil, coconut oil, and jojoba oil, which can be used to moisturize and treat different hair types. They also act as the carriers for essential oils, which are strongly concentrated oils derived from the various aromatic plants. Essential oils are very strong and can give tremendous benefits, but should always be diluted into carrier oils. They can also be used to add a wonderful aroma to whichever hair treatments you make. Here are some essential oils, carrier oils, and other valuable ingredients for hair care, all of which have been used by different cultures from around the world since before the advent of modern hair care:

- **Rosemary:** One of my personal favorite hair care ingredients, rosemary is native to the Mediterranean part of the world, where it has long been used to promote hair growth and improve scalp health. Add a few drops of rosemary essential oil to a home-made hair mask or conditioner. Alternatively, you can make a rosemary infusion from the herb itself, and use it as a hair rinse.

- **Peppermint:** Used since time immemorial by Egyptian and Greek cultures, peppermint soothes itchy scalp and promotes hair growth. Like rosemary, you can use either the essential oil (mixed into a carrier oil) or make a peppermint infusion from the herb itself.

- **Lavender:** One of the most soothing and versatile herbs known to man, lavender is particularly good to counteract stress-related hair loss. Use its essential oil, or make a herb infusion in either water or oil.

- **Tea tree oil:** The tea tree plant is native to Australia. It has long been used for hair and skin care due to its antimicrobial properties and ability to prevent and treat infections and irritations of any kind.

- **Aloe vera:** The gel of this plant (and other aloe plants, although aloe vera is most easily harvested) protects against sun damage, soothes scalp irritation, and promotes healthy hair growth. I keep an aloe in my garden, where I can easily harvest a plant and squeeze out the gel whenever necessary, but the gel can also be purchased from any pharmacy or health shop.

- **Almond oil:** This oil has gentle antimicrobial properties and works as a very gentle carrier oil for stronger essential oils. It contributes to hair shine and can be used regularly without causing the scalp to become excessively oily (although it should be rinsed off after use).

- **Jojoba oil:** Because jojoba oil is chemically similar to our own sebum, it is a very good carrier oil for scalps that tend to become too oily, helping the body regulate its own sebum production and simultaneously nourishing the hair.

Recipe: Lavender Stress-Relief Scalp Massage Oil

Scalp massages are some of the most nourishing and follicle-stimulating remedies for stressed, thinning, or alkaline scalps. If your hair is struggling, then I suggest you begin to incorporate regular scalp massages, working the oil into your skin and massaging gently with your fingertips until your entire head feels enlivened. This lavender massage oil is one of the many oils you could make—experiment with other essential oils if you'd like, as long as you remember to use a carrier oil as well.

Ingredients:

- 2 tbsp almond oil (or more, if you have very thick hair)

- 5 drops lavender essential oil

- 3 drops rosemary essential oil

- 2 drops tea tree essential oil

Instructions:

- Mix the almond oil with other essential oils of your choosing, making sure that everything is well-blended.

- Warm the mixture slightly in a double boiler, or heat it in the microwave for a few seconds.

- Part your hair into sections to make it easier to apply the oil equally, and add a few drops to your scalp.

- Rub the oil in gently, adding more if you find that there are sections of your scalp that remain dry. Continue massaging your scalp for about 5-10 minutes.

- Leave the oil on your scalp for as long as you think is necessary, anywhere between half an hour and overnight. After that, wash your hair thoroughly with a gentle shampoo.

Recipe: Rosemary and Aloe Vera Hair Mask

This soothing hair mask is easy to make and uses common ingredients, making it perfect for regular application, particularly if your scalp is irritated or your hair needs some enlivening. You can also add some yogurt to this blend, particularly if your hair needs some extra protein. If your hair is very long or thick, then multiply the quantities listed below by two to ensure you have enough to cover all your hair.

Ingredients:

- 2 tbsp rosemary leaves

- 3 tbsp aloe vera gel

- 1 tbsp coconut oil

- 3-4 drops of any essential oil of your choice

Instructions:

- Using a blender, mix all the ingredients together until they form a smooth paste.

- Apply the mask to your hair and scalp, massaging it gently into your roots. Continue massaging for a few minutes to encourage blood circulation.

- Leave the mask on for about 45 minutes.

- Wash your hair thoroughly with a gentle shampoo, preferably in lukewarm water, and follow up with a conditioner.

The two recipes discussed here are just meant to offer you a glimpse into what is possible when you begin experimenting with simple, nutritious ingredients and essential oils. Play with different ideas, making herbal rinses, hair masks, and deep-conditioning treatments that specifically suit your hair type.

You know best what you need, so lean into your innate self-awareness and get creative.

Chapter 2:

Glowing Complexion:

Unleashing the Holistic Power

of Your Face and Skin

Skincare, like hair care, can be a thorny issue for many of us. We present our faces to the world every day, using our facial expressions, eye contact, and language to relate to others. When we don't feel confident about our skin, this can have a significant impact on how it feels to relate to others, and even to look into the mirror. This is why the skincare industry is so massive—health and beauty companies know that it deeply matters to us, as both people and consumers.

If you've ever had an acne flare-up, a rash, or inexplicably dry or oily skin (and who among us hasn't?), then you know how bewildering the range of store products can be, each promising a miraculous transformation. All of them, of course, carry a hefty price tag, but to many of us the price feels justified for the promise of radiant skin it beckons. But which skincare products to choose? If marketing companies are to be believed, then we need to use a toner, cleanser, day cream, night cream, and eye cream on the daily. On top of that, specialized products such as masks and salves are advertised as the ultimate cure for a variety of ailments. Not only does this long list of products quickly become astonishingly expensive, but it can also become quite the chore to keep up with a beauty routine this complicated. Many of these products also come with a hidden cost: a long list of chemicals that we unknowingly expose our bodies to. Did you know that something as simple as a mass-made bar of soap contains, at least, a dozen different synthetic chemicals, including synthetic detergents, hardeners, and emulsifiers? (Bare-Soaps, 2016.) This realization has led many individuals, myself included, to embrace a more natural and holistic approach to skin care. By opting for natural alternatives, we can minimize our exposure to potentially harmful substances and allow our skin to breathe freely.

A holistic approach also extends beyond topical applications and dives into the realm of nourishment, movement, and self-awareness. Taking a holistic approach means looking at something as a whole, rather than focusing on isolated parts. This involves understanding that our skin is not an isolated entity, but intricately connected to our overall health and wellbeing. For example, to truly care for our skin holistically, we must address not only external factors, but also internal ones. Among other things, our diet plays a crucial role in skin health, with certain nutrients supporting skin rejuvenation and radiance. Balancing hormones, ensuring restful sleep, and practicing stress reduction techniques also contribute to a healthy complexion. A weakened immune system can manifest as skin flare-ups, emphasizing the interplay between our internal health and skin condition. By focusing on bolstering our immune system through proper nutrition, stress management, and healthy lifestyle choices, we create a strong foundation for radiant skin.

A close friend of mine once struggled for years with an inexplicable rash on her cheeks, which would flare up seemingly without rhyme or reason. After trying every skincare product she could think of, she decided to take a closer look at her diet instead. She did this by taking notes of what she had eaten every time her skin became irritated. She soon discovered that her rash became particularly active when her immune system was low, combined with eating highly processed or sugary foods. Once she realized this, she was able to focus on strengthening her gut health and on cutting out most sugar from her diet; her flare-ups soon disappeared entirely. While it can feel like more of an effort to track your body's responses in this way, over time this approach becomes much simpler and cheaper than applying copious amounts of topical products, and it offers the added benefit of improving your attunement to your own body.

In the realm of holistic skin care, knowledge is power. Understanding the unique needs of our skin, and being attuned to its signals, allows us to tailor our routines accordingly. No two individuals have identical skin, and by listening to our skin's messages, we can provide it with the care it craves. By embracing natural alternatives and adopting a holistic approach, we empower ourselves to create a harmonious relationship between our skin, body, and mind. In the following sections, we will delve deeper into specific practices, ingredients, and techniques that will guide you on your holistic skin care journey.

Simple Practices for Radiant Skin

Before taking a deeper look at nutrition and at natural skincare products, let's understand some simple holistic practices to develop radiant skin. These can be applied regardless of your skin type, genetic heritage, and circumstances, and are beneficial for your entire self, rather than just your skin.

- **Less is more.** "Under a microscope, the skin looks like a coral reef," writes physician Zach Bush (Bush, 2020).

What he means by this is that the skin, the largest organ of our body, is very much like an ecosystem of its own. It is teeming with life, not only because thousands of blood vessels provide it with nutrients and oxygen, but also because it is covered with a multitude of bacteria. It can be a bit strange to think about this, but most bacteria are good, actually—they help protect and nourish our skins, breaking down nutrients into smaller parts, and contributing to the wellbeing of our entire system. We need our skin microbiome to be teeming with a wide variety of bacteria, as well as with natural oils that further protect us. Using too many skincare products affects both the microbial life and the production of sebum. For example, using harsh antibacterial soap has a similar effect on your skin as antibiotics have on your gut—it exterminates all bacterial life, leaving the door wide open for harmful microbes to establish themselves, and leaving your body unprotected.

I find that when it comes to skin care, a good motto is "when in doubt, leave it out." Try to focus on buying products with fewer, more natural, ingredients. Look for handmade soap from local crafters, buy moisturizers from environment-friendly companies, or just make your own. This book will provide you with some recipes, with numerous more available online, as long as you use your discretion.

- **Notice your body's unique needs and patterns.** In the example I gave about my friend with the inexplicable rash, she discovered the cause of her problems by tracking her diet and her skin flare-ups. I would strongly encourage you to do the same, even if you are not struggling with any particular skin issues. How does your skin respond to different climates, to what you are eating, to exercise and sleep, or lack thereof? You may think that you know all these things already, but you might be surprised by what you discover when you start making a point of actually paying more conscious attention. It is also worth paying attention to your genetic heritage: Does your skin take after one of your parents in particular? How have your parents and other family members aged? This will give you some clues about what might be in store for you, and how to avoid some of the issues that they have encountered.

- **Keep it local.** Whenever possible, try to buy skincare products that have been locally sourced. This is, of course good, for the environment and contributes to a more holistic way of life, but it is also actually good for your skin and gut microbiomes. This is because these products contain microbes (which are found on absolutely everything) that are similar to your own, thus supporting your body's efforts to build up healthy colonies of beneficial microbes. Furthermore, herbs, oils, and other products that have been locally sourced have had to go through a less intensive shipping process, meaning that they are fresher, contain more vitamins such as vitamin C which may evaporate over time, and have fewer additives and preservatives.

- **Stay hydrated.** This sounds like obvious advice, but it may entail a bit more than you may realize at first. Dehydration really means to develop a deficit in certain salts that the body requires, most notably sodium, potassium, and magnesium. Without these, your body will struggle to retain water, regardless of how many glasses you drink per day. And, of course, prolonged dehydration has a drastic effect on the skin, lessening elasticity and vitality. To prevent this, try to become aware of how much or little water you are drinking every day. Do you often feel thirsty, even though you drink a lot of water? You may have a mineral deficiency, which is easily solved by adding some minerals to your water.

My favorite way to rehydrate my body is to add a quarter teaspoon of Himalayan salt (which contains sodium), a quarter teaspoon of cream of tartar (containing potassium), and a very small amount of Epsom salts (containing magnesium) to a glass of water once a day. If that sounds a bit salty for you, add some lemon juice as well, or take your daily salts as a shot instead of dissolved into a full glass of water.

Radiant Nutrition: Eating for Healthy Skin

Another part of our bodies which teems with microbial life is our digestive system. The concept of good gut health (which means the presence of a vibrant community of good microbes) has gained more popularity in recent years, and for all good reasons—scientists have found that the gut truly is the seat of whole-body health (Enders, 2015). And the health of our skin is directly impacted by the health of our gut—this is known as the gut-skin axis. Research has shown that the gut microbiome has a significant impact on skin diseases such as psoriasis and eczema (Thye et al., 2022), and on skin inflammation in general. If you have ever needed to take a round of antibiotics only to find your skin suddenly breaking out as a result, then you've likely experienced this yourself.

It can be disquieting to realize that your digestive system has such a significant impact, but, on the other hand, taking care of one's gut can be much less mysterious than trying to solve skin issues with a host of complicated topical applications. Our guts are also largely responsible for hormone regulation, playing a role in the production of almost every hormone we need for daily functioning, including our sex hormones (including testosterone, estrogen and progesterone) and our stress hormones (adrenaline and cortisol). Both these families of hormones have a significant influence on our skin as well. If you find that your skin is affected by stress, or that you tend to have skin outbreaks, then ensuring that your gut is as healthy as possible is also a good and sustainable solution.

Ideally, our digestive tracts should contain a vast variety of beneficial microbes which we can build up in a variety of ways. The chapter on nutrition will cover this in more depth, but for now, it would suffice to say that fermented foods—including sauerkraut, kefir, yogurt, kombucha, and even sourdough bread and red wine—help to colonize our guts with healthy bacteria. If you struggle to enjoy fermented foods, then taking a daily probiotic supplement may also work for you, although ingesting bacteria in their more natural form through food is more beneficial. Whichever approach you choose, simply keep in mind that the more varied the microbial life in our guts, the stronger our immune systems, and the more radiant our skins will be.

Another simple approach to gut health is to eat unprocessed foods from a wide variety of food groups. Try to eat foods of different colors as well, as many colors signify the presence of different antioxidants—for instance, the orange color of carrots signal the presence of beta-carotene, an important form of vitamin A. If your plate is regularly filled with leafy greens, starchy vegetables, organically-produced meat, healthy fats, herbs and spices, and fruit, then you are probably doing it right. If this isn't the case for you, then set small goals for yourself, such as trying to include one or two vegetables more per day, or eating from a food group that you don't normally include in your meals. The goal here isn't perfection, but to become attuned to what your body needs and what it is *subtly* asking for. The more you pay attention to these intricacies, the more obvious your body's responses will become, but the process should be a joyful one, rather than a guilt-filled endeavor to be healthier.

Skin-Friendly Foods

There are particular kinds of food that specifically benefit the skin. Trying to focus on eating enough of these may be a good approach for you.

- **Foods rich in omega-3 and omega-6 fatty acids:** These two fatty acids contribute significantly to skin health by keeping the skin supple, preventing it from thinning, and working against inflammation. If your skin tends to be dry or is aging faster than you'd like, then these fatty acids are absolutely essential for you. A good source of these fatty acids is flaxseed oil, which you can drizzle directly over your food or use to make a salad dressing. Fatty fish, such as salmon, herring, anchovies, and trout, are also a good source of fatty acids, although here I would add that it's best to try to source these fish locally, given the harm caused by overfishing and the resulting depletion of our natural systems. As an added bonus, fish contains a lot of zinc which is particularly good for the skin and the regulation of hormones.

- **Avocados:** Especially if you can buy them in the right season, avocados are incredibly nutritious, providing a good dose of healthy fats plus vitamins E and C, which are both essential for healthy skin.

- **Sunflower seeds:** These contain a host of skin-friendly nutrients, including zinc and vitamin E. My favorite way of eating sunflower seeds is by sprouting them and adding them to my salads as microgreens, but they can also be lightly grilled and added to other foods. Other nuts and seeds are also very good for you—however, try to soak any nuts and seeds in water for, at least, a few hours before consuming them, since this makes their nutrients more bioavailable.

- **Foods containing beta-carotene:** Vitamin A is an important antioxidant for skin health, and therefore foods high in beta-carotene—such as sweet potatoes, carrots and tomatoes—should make frequent appearances on your plate.

- **Broccoli and other plants in the cabbage family:** Cabbage and broccoli, as well as other related plants such as cauliflower and kale, may well and truly be called everyday superfoods. These plants contain a host of vitamins and minerals, as well as other components known as sulforaphane, which helps protect the skin.

- **Tomatoes:** "A tomato a day keeps the doctor away," is how I think the old adage should really go. Tomatoes are wonderful sources of various vitamins, including lutein, vitamin C, beta-carotene, and vitamin K. Personally, I try to keep a box of cherry tomatoes in my house at all times, regularly popping one or two tomatoes into my mouth as I walk past. Eating them like a small and delicious fruit is an easy option—there is no need to always make complicated salads to ensure our daily intake of veggies.

Dark chocolate, red grapes, berries, green tea, and bell peppers, as well as other colorful and fragrant foods and drinks, all greatly benefit the skin as well. Eat widely, eat with gusto, but avoid processed foods where possible, and the odds are, you'll be eating food that is good for your skin.

Topical Skin Care

Now that we've looked at how to nourish our skin from the inside out, it is time to focus on what is, according to me, the most fun part of skin care: Playing with a variety of natural ingredients to create our very own topical skincare treatments. The focus here is on all-natural, plant-based aids, many of which can also be used for other aspects of healthy living. Let's explore some of our options.

Nature's Pharmacy: Plant-Based Skincare Ingredients

There is a myriad of natural resources available to us, particularly if we make a point of noticing our environments and using the herbs and ingredients found locally. The list below is by no means exhaustive, although it's a good start, and I encourage you to pay attention to other herbs, and even foods and oils, you could use. For instance, if you have a basil plant growing on a windowsill, then infusing some boiling water with basil and using that as a gentle toner could work very well. The point is to use what is available, as long as it is backed by research. Here are some ancient healing ingredients to get you started:

- **Turmeric:** Turmeric has been used medicinally by various cultures across the world for as long as written records exist—and probably even before that. In particular, it features strongly in ancient Chinese and other Asian healing traditions, and no wonder, because turmeric is one of the most versatile and potent anti-inflammatory ingredients available to mankind. Turmeric is a root, resembling ginger, although more brightly orange, and it can be used either freshly grated or in dried form, to lessen inflammation and brighten complexion. However, take note that the active healing ingredient in turmeric, called curcumin, is activated by compounds found specifically in black pepper, so when using turmeric, make sure to add some freshly ground black pepper to your mixture for best results. My favorite way of using turmeric is to boil some turmeric powder with a bit of water on the stove, add some black pepper and allow it to turn into a paste. The paste can be added to food or used topically on the skin.

- **Green tea**: Green tea has been used medicinally in East Asia for many centuries, and once discovered by the West, it soon gained popularity all across the world. Not only does it work wonderfully as a revitalizing beverage, but it also contains various antioxidants that work wonders on the skin. It also has the ability to gently protect the skin against UV damage. You may also use it as a gentle skin toner.

- **Rosehip oil**: Rosehip is the small, greenish fruit of the rose plant, ignored by many of us in favor of the rose flower itself; however, its oil is a potent anti-aging and deeply moisturizing aid. Various South and Central American cultures have known this and used it for centuries, but nowadays rosehip oil has become popular amongst the rest of the world as well. It works effectively as a skin healer, gentle anti-inflammatory, and as an aid in reducing scars.

- **Jojoba oil:** Jojoba oil is remarkably similar to sebum in terms of pH and consistency, making it particularly good at assisting the body in regulating its own oil production. For this reason, and the fact that it is so gentle and can be used for both hair and skin, it has long been used by indigenous cultures from Mexico and

North America, which is where the jojoba plant originally sprang from.

- **Aloe:** We have already discussed the aloe plant in Chapter 1, but it is worth noting that the gel from both aloe ferox and aloe vera, as well as most other aloe plants, is an incredibly useful aid in skincare. It is often used for skin irritations, to protect from sun damage, or to heal any inflammation. Consider keeping an aloe plant in a pot and harvest the gel yourself by peeling open a leaf and cutting out the gel found inside.

- **Witch Hazel:** This plant extract is usually sold in liquid form and can be applied directly to the skin. It has historically been used by various cultures to tighten and tone the skin, working also particularly well against inflammation and acne.

Recipe: Green Tea and Witch Hazel Facial Toner

This gentle toner works well on most skin types and can be used to tone and protect skin in the morning and evening. You could also keep a small spritzer bottle of this in your purse, and refresh your skin throughout the day as necessary. Add a bit of rose water for extra rejuvenating effects, or even a teaspoon of aloe gel for extra skin nutrition.

Ingredients:

- 1 cup distilled water

- 1 green tea bag

- 1 tbsp witch hazel

- 5 drops of lavender essential oil (or gentle essential oil of your choice—rose geranium, ylang-ylang, and clary sage are also good choices)

Instructions:

- Bring the distilled water to a boil, and steep the tea bag in it for about 10 minutes.

- Remove the tea bag and allow the tea to cool down to room temperature.

- Add the witch hazel, essential oil, and other optional ingredients. Stir well.

- Keep the mixture in a clean, airtight container.

To use:

Apply the toner directly to your cleaned skin with a cotton pad. Gently pat your skin dry, or allow the toner to air dry on your skin for a few minutes. Follow with a moisturizer.

Recipe: Turmeric Face Mask

This face mask works wonderfully as an anti-inflammatory skin purifier, gently cleansing skin while soothing any skin irritations. Honey is a potent antimicrobial, and yogurt nourishes the skin, while turmeric will do some deep skin healing, permeating through into the inner layers of your skin. Turmeric does temporarily stain everything it touches yellow, so don't use this mask just before you are about to go out—use it early in the morning instead, or perhaps shortly before bedtime. Also, particularly if you suspect that you may have any skin sensitivities, do a patch test before applying the mask to your whole face for the first time.

Ingredients:

- 1 tbsp turmeric powder

- 1 tbsp honey

- 1 tbsp yogurt

- 3 drops of a gentle essential oil (such as lavender, tea tree, or rose geranium) (optional)

Instructions:

- Mix the turmeric, yogurt, honey and essential oil in a small bowl until they form a sticky paste.

- Apply the paste evenly on your face, leaving the eye area open.

- Leave the mask on for about 15 minutes, or until it becomes somewhat flaky.

- Rinse off the mask with lukewarm water—remember that any lingering yellow color will disappear within a few hours.

- Follow with a toner and gentle moisturizer.

Because all its ingredients are so gentle, you may use this mask as regularly as you'd like. I recommend trying it once a week for a few weeks to begin noticing its long-term effects.

Using food to make skincare ingredients isn't only fun; it is also surprisingly effective, since the skin absorbs nutrients just like the gut does. In other words, what's good for the belly can also be good for the skin. This turmeric face mask is one such food-based recipe, but feel free to explore other options, too. All of the ingredients listed in this chapter can work wonders on the skin, of course when matched with the right skin and co-ingredients. Combine herbs, oils, essential oils, and spices to make cleansers, masks, and even to moisturize your skin. The ingredients discussed in some of the next chapters, particularly those focused on organ health, can often be used on the skin as well. As long as you choose your ingredients wisely and do a patch test before using your home-made treatment for the first time, you are sure to conjure up wonderful, tailor-made recipes.

Chapter 3:

Serenity Unleashed:

Harmonizing Your Neck and

Shoulders Through Holistic

Practices

If ever you go on a hike along a mountainous region, or even on a stroll next to a river or in a forest, you'll immediately notice the impact time has had on that place: How trees have grown and vied for space among each other, how rocks have fallen, and how water has paved a way through ravines. Everything is a delicate interplay between different forces, leaving an indelible mark upon the landscape. In the same way, the human body is also a landscape. In the same way that a piece of land holds stories, our bodies hold everything that has ever happened to us, and treasures the story of our responses to all external and internal events.

The neck and shoulders are some of the most telling parts of our bodies, soaking up the strain that we unconsciously experience throughout our lives. Along with our hands, feet, and hips, the neck and shoulders are one of the sites that usually hold the most trauma, both physical and emotional.

Concurrently, healing neck and shoulder pain can unlock tremendous physical and emotional healing for our entire selves. Learning to attune to the messages our upper bodies are sending to us is an important part of holistic wellness.

Understanding Neck and Shoulder Tension

All of us have, at one time or another, must have experienced neck or shoulder pain. Particularly in our westernized society, most of us spend large portions of time working on our computers or mobile phones, which isn't what our bodies have evolved to do. That, and the fact that we tend to sit for longer periods of time than what is deemed healthy, already leads to various forms of tension in our upper back bodies. On top of that, as I've mentioned, our neck and shoulders are points where many of us store stress. We react to stressors by tensing our necks, by lifting our shoulders, by tightening our entire bodies and moving less than what is actually necessary. All of these things have a cumulative impact.

However, everybody is different, and the ways that you may experience neck and shoulder pain or tension are (or can be) different from anyone else's. For that reason, when discussing upper back body issues, it is necessary to practice some bodily self-awareness. To that end, here are a few questions you could ask yourself:

- Where, in your upper back body, do you habitually tense up? Do you have certain areas or muscle groups that routinely ache while doing repetitive tasks, or while experiencing stress?

- Do you feel different kinds of aches depending on the stressors? For example, there is a spot on my upper back, just to the right of my spine, which starts aching when I've been on my computer for too long. This is different from the ache I feel in my neck when I'm stressed or worried, or from the knots that form in my left shoulder after experiencing interrupted sleep. Try to draw up a "pain map" of sorts for your upper back body, either in your mind's eye or actually on paper. Where are those painful spots? Which kinds of circumstances make them tense up?

- How does your habitual upper back body tension feel? Do you feel as if there is a tight band of pain across your shoulders? Do you have painful knots in your neck and along your spine? Is it a creeping kind of pain, which gradually makes its way up your spine and eventually becomes a tension headache? Many of us deal with pain by ignoring it for as long as possible, or by swallowing a few painkillers and soldiering on, but pain is a message from the body. You don't need to be a physician or an expert diagnostician to learn to decode the messages your body is sending you every time you feel pain—simply learn to tune into what you're feeling and start recognizing it. "Ah, this is the twinge-like ache I get when I've been sitting for too long," you'll soon start saying, followed by the solution: "I should get up and do a few stretches to honor what my body is trying to tell me."

- Do you have limited movement in your back or arms? Sometimes, we don't experience upper back body pain as such, but we do gradually lose some range of motion... often without realizing it. A very common example of this is that, as most of us tend to hunch forward, we lose the ability to move our arms backward entirely. Here are a few ways to test your range of motion:

o   Sit with your back flat against a wall, making sure that your back connects with it from top to bottom. Now lift your upper arms, keeping them flat against the wall as well. Can you raise your arms at all, without moving either your arms or head away from the wall? If not, then the area between your shoulders, where the neck connects with the rest of the spine, has become tight.

o   Move your head slowly down. Are you able to rest your chin on your chest? Similarly, try to rest each ear on each matching shoulder, resisting the urge to lift the other shoulder in response. How far can you lower your head before the other shoulder starts protesting?

o   Try to put your arms behind your back, clasp your hands together, and straighten your arms. Are you able to do this? If so, do you feel any muscle group protesting?

The goal with these simple tests is not to make you feel worried or guilty about your range of motion, or lack thereof. There is no right or wrong, and different bodies have different capabilities. However, these are the areas where you may have been ignoring your body's messages, and where you should begin to tune into. Are there any slower, gentle ways you could start untangling your knotted muscles, or moving in ways you aren't normally used to?

Holistic Techniques for Upper Back Body Tension Relief

As we've begun discussing, much of holistic healing begins with just noticing. From this point of noticing, we can become aware of the nudges our bodies are giving us, essentially cultivating a trust relationship with our own bodies. To me, it sometimes helps to imagine my body as a beloved pet: Our animals signal things to us all the time, but we have to learn to read those signs and understand what they are trying to communicate to us. If we consistently ignore what they are trying to tell us, the bond of trust and communication between ourselves and our pet will become frayed. However, it is never too late to start paying attention. The moment you decide to sit down with your pet (or child, or partner, or with your own body, for that matter) and pay attention, the relationship becomes revitalized. Quickly, far sooner than you may have otherwise thought possible, you will begin to pick up on signals you had never noticed before. To facilitate this increased noticing of your bodily signals, here are a few things you can do:

- **Cultivate acceptance of and gentleness toward your body:** Many of the messages your neck and shoulders may send you will be for small changes, or simply to draw your attention to something. If you have carried your stress or trauma in your shoulders for decades, then, for you, it is likely that a part of reinstating your relationship to your upper back body will simply involve acknowledgment of your pain, sending loving thoughts to the self who has had to carry this burden for this long, and making small postural changes. If you are comfortable with it, you could also practice sending loving thoughts toward the affected area of your neck and shoulders. Whether or not loving thoughts actually make a physical difference is a different story, but slipping into this mindset definitely brings about greater awareness of the area, which is sometimes enough to help you sit in a different position/style, take more regular breaks while working, or just push you to move more gently. This is the start of holistic pain treatment of any kind.

- **Rest:** Many of us have jobs or lifestyles that run counter to our natural rhythms, forcing us to keep up a pace of life that, if we are honest, doesn't really feel good. This doesn't mean that we should quit our jobs and go live in the woods—there are small ways through which we can begin to consciously incorporate rest into our lives. This will not only have an effect on our necks and shoulders, but also on our general health. For example, try to take a five-minute break in between large chunks of work. Depending on your cycles, and on how long you can remain focused on a single task, you may try taking a break every half-an-hour, or even more frequently than that (depending on your ability to focus). During these breaks, stretch gently, swing your arms from side to side, or bend forward and touch your toes for a moment. Try to prioritize rest in other ways too: Making sure that you go to bed early enough, that your quality of sleep is good, and that you make time for yourself during the day.

- **Examine your sleep position:** Many of us have quite bad sleep postures, often waking up with a crick in our necks or with a dead shoulder. To prevent this, first of all try to ensure that both your mattress and pillow are firm enough—memory foam cushions work particularly well for good sleep posture. If you sleep on your side, then putting a pillow between your knees can help keep your spine aligned. If you sleep on your back, then putting a pillow under your knees is also a good idea. In general, try to avoid sleeping on your stomach, since this is the posture that leads, most frequently, to back pain.

- **Monitor how long you sit:** The human body, with its long spine and various supporting muscles, was not really made for continuous sitting. Instead, we evolved to alternate positions regularly: walking, sitting, running, crouching, walking again, and lying down. Sitting for a long time means that our lower back bodies need to absorb more and more weight, which often means that our upper bodies tense and try to lift up to compensate for the weight being shifted down. To help with this, simply make a point of getting up every half an hour or so, whether you are at your desk or in front of the TV. Your body will thank you later for this little exercise.

- **Apply heat:** Contracting muscles also cause decreased blood flow to that region, frequently contributing to muscle pain. To counteract that, apply a heat pack to the painful area—this will allow the blood vessels to expand, rushing blood to the area where it can work its healing magic.

- **Posture exercises:** Especially when we spend a lot of time working on our computers, our posture often becomes compromised, leading to long-term stiffness or pain. One of the most common issues is that we slump our shoulders and jut our heads forward slightly, which eventually translates into loss of mobility in the upper spine. A simple remedy is to pull your chin in, almost as if making a double chin, and holding this pose for a few minutes before relaxing your head again.

This trains the body to hold your head in better alignment with the rest of your spine. Another useful posture exercise is to sit against a wall, making sure that your back is flat against it from the pelvis to the head. Now open your arms wide until they, too, touch the wall, and raise them slightly, holding them in this position for as long as possible. This stretches the tight back muscles on both sides of your spine. Cat-cow exercises and forward-fold stretches can also help the tightest parts of your back loosen gently.

Harnessing the Power of Nature: Natural Ingredients for Gentle Back Care

Nature provides us with various herbs and oils that can loosen sore muscles, improve blood circulation, and work gentle healing magic into the tightest of tissues. These ingredients have been used before the advent of modern medicine, and with good reason: They work and are easily available. Today we have access to ancient knowledge from all corners of the world on how to treat our bodies, allowing us the freedom to craft our own treatments. Let's look at a few important ingredients:

- **Comfrey:** This plant, often considered a weed because it grows so abundantly, has a long history of traditional use for bone and muscle support. Its leaves and roots contain allantoin, a compound known for its ability to promote cell proliferation and tissue regeneration. Comfrey should only be used topically, in the form of salve, ointments, or poultices to soothe sprains, strains, bruises, or minor fractures.

- **Eucalyptus**: Eucalyptus essential oil is renowned for its anti-inflammatory properties. It can be very beneficial in relieving muscle and joint pain caused by inflammation. Eucalyptus oil can be mixed into a carrier oil, such as coconut oil, and applied topically through massage, or a few drops could be added to a warm bath to ease muscle tension and promote relaxation.

- **Ginger:** Ginger has been used for centuries as a natural remedy for various ailments, including muscle and joint discomfort. It contains anti-inflammatory compounds which help reduce pain and swelling. Consuming ginger tea, or incorporating fresh ginger into meals, can provide much relief and support the body's natural healing processes. You can also grate raw ginger and apply it to any painful area as a compress.

- **Arnica:** Arnica is a popular herb, widely used in topical preparations for its anti-inflammatory properties. It can help alleviate muscle soreness, bruises, and sprains. Arnica gel or cream can be gently massaged onto the affected area to ease discomfort.

- **Lemongrass:** Lemongrass essential oil possesses pain-relieving and anti-inflammatory properties, thereby making it an excellent choice for relieving muscle and joint pain. Its invigorating citrusy aroma can also help uplift the mood and leave you feeling more energized. Diluted lemongrass essential oil can be applied topically, or it can be used in a diffuser for aromatherapy benefits.

- **Turmeric:** Turmeric contains a compound called curcumin which has strong anti-inflammatory and antioxidant properties. This makes turmeric particularly good at addressing muscle and joint discomfort caused by inflammation. Add turmeric to your food as often as possible (combined with black pepper which activates turmeric's healing compounds), or make a turmeric paste to use topically.

Remedy: Soothing Neck-and-Shoulder Herbal Compress

Ingredients:

- 2 tbsp dried eucalyptus leaves
- 2 tbsp ginger root, fresh or dried
- 2 tbsp dried arnica flowers
- 2 tbsp dried lemongrass leaves
- 3 tbsp dried comfrey leaves
- Cheesecloth or similar permeable cloth
- Rubber band or piece of string

Instructions:

- Put all the herbs into a blender and mix them together until they are finely chopped.

- Place the herbs in the center of your cloth, then gather the corners of the cloth together, tying it together with a rubber band or string. This should form a secured pouch with the herbs in the middle.

- Submerge the herb pouch into warm water, leaving it there until all the herbs are well-saturated.

- Remove the pouch from the warm water and squeeze out any excess water. The pouch should be warm, but not too hot.

- Sit in a comfortable position, or lie down, then place the pouch on any painful area of your body. Allow the healing compounds of the various herbs to seep through the cloth into your body, letting it sit for about 15 minutes.

- Once you've removed the pouch, gently roll your shoulder (or other affected area) to check pain and mobility, or massage the area for a while. You should feel a gentle loosening in tension.

Remedy: Eucalyptus and Peppermint Balm

Ingredients:

- ⅓ cup coconut oil

- 2 tbsp beeswax pellets

- 2 tbsp arnica oil

- 8 drops peppermint essential oil

- 12 drops eucalyptus essential oil

Instructions:

- Place a stainless-steel bowl, or double heater, over a pot of gently simmering water, then melt the coconut oil, beeswax and arnica oil together until they are blended together.

- Remove the oils from the heat and let them cool slightly, then add the essential oils. Mix everything together.

- Pour the mixture into an airtight container and allow it to cool until it becomes solidified.

- Massage about half a teaspoon of the balm into a stiff neck or shoulder, rubbing for a few minutes until the balm has permeated the skin thoroughly.

As we discovered in the previous chapters as well, there are numerous creative ways we can use natural ingredients to soothe and heal our ailments. The two recipes listed above are just two examples—try exploring different ingredients, checking in regularly with your body to feel what works or what doesn't. Your body will tell you what it needs when you begin to listen closely.

Chapter 4:

Heart's Symphony: Nurturing Holistic Harmony in Your Chest and Heart

As you will have noticed by now, we have been gently winding our way down the human body: beginning our journey with the head, the face, the neck and shoulders, and now arriving at the heart—the seat of vitality and emotion. This is the first chapter where we will be focusing on an internal organ, which means placing the focus on what happens inside of us, rather than what is visible to others. This can ask for a more subtle approach—there are no salves or oils that we can apply to our heart, and so we need to listen more deeply instead, attuning to the deeply felt ways we may look after our hearts.

Having come this far in this book, you must be aware by now that when it comes to holistic wellbeing, everything is interconnected. Our skin speaks of our internal health, our scalps reflect our hormonal histories, our back muscles tense and relax according to our lived experiences. This interrelatedness between everything becomes particularly clear when we focus on the heart, which affects every other aspect of our bodies (and even our emotions). Since time immemorial, humans have known this, and have recognized that a healthy heart is crucial for a vibrant existence. Language reflects this, too, which is why so many expressions contain the word "heart": "heartfelt," "from the heart," "knowing it off by heart," "tugging the heartstrings," "the heart of the matter," "heartsore," and so on. We know, somehow, that this brave organ, pumping oxygenated blood to every corner of our bodies, represents more than just physical survival. It speaks of our courage, our resilience, and our ability to feel deeply.

On a more tangible level, heart disease is still the leading cause of death among both men and women in the US, and in many other western countries, too, pointing to the importance of maintaining a healthy heart (Buettner, 2010). Beyond issues of life and death, a healthy heart is also important for energy and vitality—unacknowledged heart issues can make it harder to complete everyday tasks, to exercise, and to enjoy other activities that form part and parcel of our lives. However, because the heart is an internal organ, it isn't always as easy to relate to as more visible parts of the body. For instance, your skin might tell you when you have been eating something odd, when the air is too dry or damp, or when you need to change your skincare routine. But how to read the messages your heart is sending you? Well, through the rest of your body, of course. Let's take a look at some of the ways you may interpret signals from your heart:

- **Resting heart rate:** Have you ever tried checking how fast your heart beats? This is one of the most basic signifiers of heart health... and the easiest to check. Furthermore, tuning into your heartbeat and becoming familiar with your own rhythms can be a profound experience. To do this, count down a minute with a timer while counting your heartbeats, while sitting in a relaxed state. Typically, your resting heart rate should be between 60-100 beats per minute. If you are very fit, it might be lower than that, but if your resting heart rate is higher, then this might be a cause for concern. Don't worry if your heart seems to beat irregularly every now and then, though—every movement affects our heartbeats, and the gap between every beat is not necessarily the same.

- **Heart rate recovery**: Does your heart quickly return to its resting rate once you stop doing strenuous exercise? This is a sure sign of a healthy heart. If, on the other hand, you find your heart racing long after you have completed a task, or your breath remaining short well after, then your heart would benefit from some boosting.

- **Blood pressure:** Blood pressure is usually measured by a medical professional, but this doesn't mean that you need to be in dire straits to have it checked. If you are wondering about your heart or haven't checked in a long time, then going for a routine check is probably a good idea. Your blood pressure should preferably be below 120/80 mm Hg. If it is much higher, then this counts as high blood pressure. You can bring down your blood pressure with many of the approaches we will discuss in this chapter, so don't panic if yours is elevated.

- **Energy levels and breathing:** Do you feel able to cope with all the daily tasks you need to complete? A healthy heart is one that supplies enough oxygen to your entire body, allowing you to do occasionally physically strenuous tasks, to move about and engage with people without getting exhausted. If, on the other hand, you find yourself suddenly too exhausted to complete what you could have initially done easily in a day, then you might consider the possibility that your heart is sending you a message—even if it isn't a heart disease, your heart might very well be asking for some rest and acknowledgment. Similarly, if you find yourself getting out of breath after completing small tasks or walking some distance, then you should consider tuning more closely into your heart's needs.

Remember that none of these signs of heart health or ill-health are make-or-break signs, nor do they determine your fate. The holistic perspective on heart health is that there are many "whole-body things" we can do to take care of our hearts, and that it is never too late to make an improvement. Let's look at some of the practical ways through which you can begin to take gentle care of your heart:

Heart-Healthy Nutrition: Nourishing Your Cardiovascular System

When it comes to eating for a healthy heart, the good news is that food that is beneficial for your cardiovascular system is also good for the rest of your body. This is the beauty of holistic wellbeing: One healthy choice reflects across your body, and every organ simply represents a part of the bigger whole. Keep this in mind as we go through this list—the goal is not only to keep your heart healthy, but also to nourish your entire body. A robust gut biome and resplendent skin are co-advantages of making these good choices.

- **Eat more flavonoids:** In his book, *The Blue Zone* (2010), researcher Dan Buettner writes that people from a variety of long-living cultures, all across the world, have a few dietary habits in common. This points us to the possibility that eating as *they* eat, at least to some degree, would also be good for our health and longevity. One of the things many long-living people seem to eat is foods containing flavonoids. Flavonoids are a group of compounds, found naturally in many foods, which are high in antioxidants, are nutrient-dense, contain high anti-inflammatory properties, and help manage cholesterol levels. Eating foods high in flavonoids is particularly good for the heart. These foods are often naturally colorful and very flavorful, and can include grapes (and red wine), berries, onions and garlic, tomatoes, broccoli, cocoa, parsley and bell peppers.

Do you recognize some of the foods on this list? That's because many of them have already been mentioned in Chapter 2, where we discussed skin health. As I mentioned there, a good way to ensure you fill your plate with various vitamins and nutrients is by making sure that your plate is as colorful as possible. Berries, dark chocolate, tomatoes, and various leafy greens—all pack a high nutrient punch, and both your skin and heart benefit from that.

- **Consume healthy fats:** Until quite recently, most people believed that foods high in fat, especially animal fats, are particularly bad for cardiovascular health; the general recommendation was to switch to low-fat products, and to swap animal fats for vegetable oils and margarine. More and more research is now showing us that consuming fats is not necessarily a problem, although highly processed fats such as margarine may actually be detrimental to our health (Harvard Health Publishing, 2020). In fact, regularly consuming healthy fats helps keep our blood sugar low and keeps the body functioning optimally (Pelz, 2022). Avocados, mature cheeses, olive oil, flaxseed oil, and nuts and seeds are particularly good for your heart, so try incorporating those into almost every meal.

- **Cut down on sodium:** What many of us don't realize when we eat highly processed foods is that most of those foods are very high in sodium, which heightens blood pressure and is generally detrimental to heart health. To avoid this, try to eat fewer pre-packaged foods, crisps, and other processed foods. However, this doesn't mean that all salts are bad—as I discussed in some of the previous chapters, salts help us remain hydrated and form an important part of the cycling of minerals and nutrients through the body. Try adding small amounts of Epsom salts and non-iodized salt (such as Himalayan salt or rock salt) to your drinking water, and consume foods high in potassium, such as tomatoes and bananas (which happen to contain flavonoids as well, so it's a win-win situation!)

Heart-Healthy Movement

Perhaps, the best thing you can do for your heart is to move. The heart's function is to carry oxygenated blood to every part of our body, and bring back the deoxygenated blood to our lungs. By moving our bodies, we train the heart, which is also a muscle, to transport blood more efficiently, which subsequently gives us more energy, thus making movement easier—it's a very positive cycle. However, moving regularly doesn't mean you need to spend hours every day doing strenuous exercise; many of us have busy schedules and simply don't find the time to exercise as much as we would like. Feeling guilty over this is counterproductive, and also quite unnecessary, since there are simple, doable steps you can take to exercise your heart instead:

- **Make lifestyle adaptations:** Making a point to move regularly can become second nature, once you have made it a habit. For instance, when given the option, take the stairs instead of the elevator, ride a bicycle or walk to the shops instead of driving there. Plant and maintain a small garden—gardening is, surprisingly, a good exercise and offers the rewards of healthy food as well.

- **Walk:** Walking is one of the most gentle and beneficial types of exercises. It helps relax the mind, and is the one type of exercise that all healthy centenarians have in common (Buettner, 2010). It is quite gentle on the joints, which means fewer injuries, and it can be a wonderful opportunity to explore more of your neighborhood or get out in nature. I found that having a dog helped me get up and move much more regularly, so you might consider enlisting a pet's help in sticking to a walking routine—saying no to a Labrador begging for a walk is more than most of us are able to do. If having a pet isn't viable for you, then consider enlisting the help of a friend or partner who will walk with you and keep you accountable. Soon, you'll no longer even need that support, as you will start experiencing the simple joy of traversing the world by yourself.

- **Try High Intensity Interval Training:** On top of walking or other similarly gentle exercise, it is good for us to do some aerobic exercises every day as well. "Aerobic" means "contains air," pointing to the fact that faster-paced movement encourages the heart to pump oxygenated blood faster. It is good to occasionally elevate one's heart rate, training the heart muscle, and to allow the heart rate to settle again afterward. However, this doesn't mean you need to dust off your long-forgotten aerobics home training DVDs, or invest in an exercise bike. Instead, consider exploring the myriad types of High Intensity Interval Training (HIIT) routines, many of which could be found online.

These are designed to get you moving vigorously for just a few minutes, getting the blood pumping to your extremities, flushing you with heat and oxygen, before dropping you to a rest again. Doing HIIT for a few minutes at a time, a few times a day, can make a significant difference in your fitness levels and heart health.

My favorite way to do HIIT is to use a rebounder. It is a small trampoline where you can jog in one place, do silly jumps, hop to music, as well as do some squats and other forms of exercise. Because of the elasticity of the trampoline, you'll be exercising your core and balance as well, without feeling as if you are doing so. If you don't like the idea of a trampoline, you could also do jumping jacks, dance to a favorite song, or find a HIIT workout online that speaks to you.

Cultivating Emotional Wellbeing: The Heart-Mind Connection

As discussed earlier, there is a reason the heart features so prominently in our everyday language, particularly when we speak of our life force or our emotions: The heart is, indeed, more than just a life-giving muscle. It is deeply affected by our thoughts and emotions, and is consistently bound with our body in a relationship known as the heart-mind connection. You might have probably experienced how the heart can start racing simply at the thought of something terrifying happening, or in the throes of new love. Our hearts respond to a thousand tiny messages coming from the brain stem, every moment of the day, adjusting our heart rates accordingly, pumping blood to the parts of our bodies that need it the most. If you are prone to blushing, then you may know that even the act of blushing is simply a response from your heart—picking up on the sense of embarrassment flooding your body; for some unknown reason, it sends more blood to the cheeks and neck, resulting in that deep flush that so many of us can easily tell.

Did you know that it is possible to actually die of a broken heart? Though medically rare, there have been confirmed cases of heart failure being caused by extreme sadness: a medical condition called "the broken heart syndrome" (American Heart Association, 2022). This is caused when the heart responds to the surge of stress hormones that flood the body after receiving any bad news. In most cases, this is non-fatal—and you may have experienced a smaller version of this yourself, if your heart has ever constricted after hearing something sad or scary. It does illustrate quite strikingly, however, how connected the heart is to our emotions and mind.

Conversely, calming the heart rate can also calm the mind. One way to get racing, anxious thoughts under control is to slow down our breathing, which slows the heart rate, convincing our bodies that we are safe. There are various types of breathwork practices that accomplish this; in particular, research has shown that exhaling for longer than the length of the corresponding inhale can almost immediately lower the heart rate. One such simple exercise is to breathe in deeply for four counts, to hold the breath for two, then breathe out in controlled fashion for eight counts, and hold the breath for two counts again. Repeating this a few times is an immediately effective way of calming the heart rate. If you are looking for a more enlivening type of breathwork, then controlled breathing linked to time can also be a good option. Try breathing out for five seconds, then breathing out for five seconds as well, matching the length of your inhale exactly. Repeat this for a few minutes until your body begins feeling calm.

Ancient Wisdom: Natural Ingredients for Heart Health

When it comes to maintaining a healthy heart, nature provides us with an array of ingredients that have been treasured for centuries for their cardiovascular benefits. Since we are almost halfway through this book, you'll begin to see a few superstar ingredients popping up again and again—many of the ingredients listed below are also beneficial to the skin, the hair, and to the health of other organs—which becomes yet another example of the innately holistic nature of nature's healing. Let's explore some of these ingredients and how they can be used to support heart health:

- **Hawthorn:** Hawthorn is a herb known for its beneficial effects on cardiovascular health. It contains flavonoids, antioxidants, and other compounds that can help improve blood flow, strengthen the heart muscle, and support overall cardiovascular function. Hawthorn can be consumed as a tea, or in supplement form, to promote heart health and regulate blood pressure.

- **Garlic:** Garlic has been used for centuries in various cultures for its medicinal properties. It contains sulfur compounds which have been shown to support heart health by promoting healthy blood circulation, reducing blood pressure, and improving cholesterol levels. Incorporating fresh garlic into meals or even taking garlic supplements can help harness its cardiovascular benefits.

- **Turmeric:** We have met turmeric several times now, and, trust me, this isn't the last list it will feature on. Because turmeric is such a strong anti-inflammatory agent, it can effectively counteract oxidative stress and inflammation in the body, thus supporting the heart in its optimal functioning.

- **Cayenne Pepper**: Cayenne pepper contains capsaicin, a compound responsible for both its spicy taste and potential cardiovascular benefits. Capsaicin has been found to support heart health by improving blood circulation, reducing blood pressure, and supporting healthy cholesterol levels.

- **Flaxseed Oil:** Flaxseed oil is rich in omega-3 fatty acids, specifically alpha-linolenic acid (ALA), which can help reduce inflammation, support healthy blood vessels, and maintain optimal heart function. Add cold-pressed flaxseed oil to salad dressings and smoothies, or simply take a few sips every day to maintain excellent heart health.

Recipe: Garlic and Hawthorn Tonic

This simple tonic is easy to make and tastes surprisingly delicious, especially if you enjoy the pungency of garlic. Drink this as often as you'd like, and try adding different herbs every time, experiment with different flavors to accompany the garlic and hawthorn.

Ingredients:

- 2 medium cloves of garlic, crushed or finely chopped

- 2 tsp dried hawthorn berries

- 1 and a ½ cup drinking water

- Fresh or dried herbs according to your taste—holy basil, thyme and rosemary work well, among others

- A few drops of freshly squeezed lemon juice (optional)

Instructions:

- Bring the water to a boil in a small saucepan.

- Add the garlic, hawthorn berries and herbs, and let them simmer over low heat for roughly 20 minutes, or until the water is at the volume of about one cup.

- Remove from the heat, and strain the liquid into a cup. Once the liquid has cooled down a bit, add lemon juice. Drink and enjoy!

Recipe: Turmeric Golden Milk

A much-loved drink in many parts of the world, golden milk can work as a wonderful substitute for coffee, or as a calming and restorative drink before bedtime. If you are using a creamy plant milk, such as coconut milk, then keep in mind that the drink can be very rich, so consider diluting it with some water (if your stomach is quite sensitive):

Ingredients:

- 1 and a ½ cup milk or plant milk

- 1 tsp ground turmeric

- ⅓ teaspoon ground cinnamon

- Pinch of black pepper

- Pinch of nutmeg (optional)

- ½ tsp grated ginger

- Honey, to taste

Instructions:

- Heat the milk over very low heat, watching it closely to prevent it from reaching boiling point.

- Stir in the rest of the ingredients, then whisk the mixture thoroughly until they are well blended into the milk.

- Remove from heat and consume immediately.

Making a point to incorporate simple, healthy ingredients into your diet, and adding small extras such as golden milk and tonics benefits your heart tremendously—and it's not the only organ that will be thanking you. Right next to the heart lies the stomach, part of a system just as important as the heart itself:

the digestive system. What's good for the heart is good for the belly, too, more often than not, as we'll see in the coming chapter, wherein we'll investigate the ins and outs of the digestive system.

Chapter 5:

Digestive Vitality: Unlocking the Synergy of Holistic Wellness in Your Digestive System

Situated next to and below the heart lies the digestive system—an equally important yet more complex, life-giving group of organs responsible not only for processing food, but also for immunity, nervous system regulation, and hormone regulation.

In everyday language, we often use the metaphor of the heart as the seat of our emotions: The organ responsible for our deepest and most vulnerable feelings. As we saw in the previous chapter, there is actually some truth to that, since the heart does respond to every emotional fluctuation, and correspondingly help regulate our feelings. Similarly, we often refer to the gut as the center of our consciousness and courage—phrases like "gut feeling," "gut-wrenching," "it takes guts," "a fire in your belly," and "I can't stomach them" show how we intuitively understand that our digestive systems are somehow relevant to our deepest experiences of intuition and knowledge. As much as we feel emotions in our chests, we also feel them in our bellies. Experiencing a hollow sense of dread, a full sense of contentment, or having butterflies before doing something exciting—these are a few things that we all have felt at some point in our lives, haven't we?

So, how does the gut work and what causes this variety of feelings in our digestive system? And, if the gut is so complex and important, how can we best take care of it to ensure that we live with vibrancy? Well, first it is important to understand what exactly the gut is. Sometimes, people refer to it as a single organ, but it is really made up of different organs, all forming one long, interconnected system. The mouth, teeth and tongue, together with a few digestive enzymes and beneficial bacteria, already begin the digestive process, after which food travels down the esophagus and reaches the stomach. The stomach is located behind the heart and lungs, in the lower part of the chest cavity. It is pouch-shaped, which allows for liquids to pass through directly into the small intestine, while more solid food stays behind in the stomach, where it is further digested with the help of strong stomach acids and the churning of our strong stomach muscles.

Once ready, the food then passes through into the small intestine, which is a long tube folded many times over to allow it to fit into our abdomen. If straightened, the small intestine can be about three to six yards long. It is also full of small protrusions called villi. All of these villi tremendously increase the surface area of our intestines—if we were to fold out and straighten all the villi in our intestines, their length altogether would be about five miles! The reason we need this much surface area is so that the food we have eaten can come into maximal contact with digestive enzymes and absorbent surfaces, where the different nutrients are broken into smaller components and successfully absorbed into the body. After that, the food remnants move into the large intestine, and ultimately the colon which is the last part of the large intestine from where the leftover portions are finally excreted. The story of digestion is one of the most remarkably thorough processes in our bodies, with every bacterium, intestinal fold, stomach acids and enzymes playing independent, crucial roles. Protecting the integrity of this process, and making sure that we maintain a good balance of healthy bacteria and enzymes, is crucial for our continued wellbeing, as it affects every other aspect of our bodies and minds. Let's take a closer look at some of the ways in which we can begin supporting our digestive system.

Go With Your Gut: Supporting Your Gut Microbiome

In the small intestine we begin to see increasing populations of microbes, but this isn't where they are found the most, since remnants of stomach acid prevent many colonies of bacteria from flourishing here. However, once the food moves into the large intestine, we begin to see a massive increase in bacterial life, with as many as 300 to 1,000 types of bacteria living here. These microbes are tremendously important to our digestive system—although most of the macronutrients (proteins, fats and carbs) are processed in our small intestine, more of the magic happens in the large intestine. Substances that have not been processed before are now broken down by these bacteria, providing the body with essential fatty acids and vitamins. These microbes also help sharpen our immune system, and produce and regulate different hormones. When people mention the "gut microbiome," they are really speaking about the complex system of bacteria living here, and the innumerable functions they fulfill. For instance, did you know that 90% of the body's serotonin—also known as the "feel-good hormone"—is made in the gut (Enders, 2015; Cummings,

2017)? Not only that, but when the gut microbiome is weakened or comprises few types of bacteria, it can lead to autoimmune diseases, allergic reactions, mental illnesses, and even obesity. The good news is that almost all our ailments can, at least, be improved by simply improving the health of our gut biome. Keeping that in mind, let's take a look at some of the ways you can help your gut-flora thrive:

- **Eat fermented foods:** We spoke about this shortly in previous chapters, but it's worth repeating: Fermented foods are some of the most important sources of beneficial and vibrant bacteria you could possibly consume. Food fermentation is a preservation process that has been used by humans for millennia—sailors even ate sauerkraut (fermented cabbage) aboard ships to prevent scurvy! Fermented foods not only contain high numbers of beneficial bacteria, but they are also very high in nutrients—fermented vegetables can contain exponentially more vitamins than their freshly picked counterparts, for instance. Furthermore, many fermented foods are also high in fiber, which is very beneficial for the functioning of the large intestine. If you are not used to eating fermented foods, then you could take a smaller step—buy an interesting-looking beetroot ferment or sauerkraut from your local farmer's market, and see what you like. Even a few small bites every day can make a large difference. Keep in mind that there are many ferments to choose from; one will surely strike your fancy. If none work for you, regularly using a probiotic supplement may also benefit you.

- **Eat prebiotics:** While fermented foods fall under the category of probiotics, prebiotics are equally important, and often go unnoticed. Prebiotics are basically any food type containing different kinds of fiber that the human body cannot easily digest. The fiber is thus passed down to the large intestine, where beneficial bacteria can feast on it. Most harmful bacteria in the body are not able to digest prebiotics, so adding these to your diet ensures that the colonies of beneficial bacteria in your gut consistently outnumber the harmful ones, growing strong of their diet of roughage. Foods high in prebiotics include plants in the onion family, starches such as potatoes and rice, and fibrous vegetables. Highly processed food, such as pasta and white bread, contains far less fiber which is why they are so non-nutritious to the body.

- **Use antibiotics cautiously:** Antibiotics are extremely useful and even life-saving in many circumstances, but they do work according to a rather harsh system: They kill most of the bacteria in your body, thus eliminating all harmful ones, but taking many of the good ones along, too. Especially if your immune system is already compromised, this can have a long-lasting effect on your digestive system. To avoid that, be judicious about using antibiotics—if at all possible, try to use natural or less harsh remedies, and only make use of antibiotics when other medicines are not working.

- **Take small actions**: There are many small steps that can make a massive difference in your gut health. One of these is to try adopting a diet that is as varied as possible. Different bacteria specialize in digesting different foods, which means that eating from a large food group feeds many different bacteria. Incorporate herbs and spices into your diet, add different types of leaves to your salads, and consume a few types of good oils every day, even if in much smaller quantities. Foods containing flavonoids, which we discussed in the section on heart health, are also particularly good for your gut, so be sure to eat them as frequently as possible.

The Mind-Gut Connection

As we have seen, protecting and helping our gut microbiome to thrive is essential for continued health. However, microbes aren't the only noteworthy role players in the story of our digestive system. Our stomach and intestinal tract are also surprisingly rich in nerve endings, picking up on messages inside the gut and responding accordingly throughout the day. The stomach also responds to messages coming from elsewhere in the body, and, in fact, the brain and gut are connected to each other through the vagus nerve, one of the largest nerves in the body. You could say that the gut and brain have a direct line of communication, which allows them to respond and adapt to each other at all times.

Research has proven that the digestive tract has a direct impact on various areas of the brain, including those responsible for fight-or-flight responses, for decision-making, and for the regulation of emotions such as joy and fear (Enders, 2015). This means that your emotions will necessarily impact your digestion and vice versa. Many of us know this to be true from experience—have you ever suffered from a "nervous stomach"? This term is often used for people who experience regular sensations of churning, cramping, tightness, indigestion, nausea, and gassiness due to emotional stress. This is because of the aforementioned brain-gut connection. Fortunately, this also means that supporting your digestive system can help calm any emotional distress you may be experiencing. Since the gut is responsible for most of our serotonin production, as well as many other hormones, it is especially important to ensure that it is well taken care of. Giving your gut the support it needs during a bout of indigestion will mean that your stomach sends signals of wellness to your brain, where the "state of emergency" is called off and your emotions begin settling.

Sometimes, however, trying to calm your belly in order to calm your mind just doesn't work. A harmful cycle can be set in motion, where the stomach produces more acid because of the stress messages it receives. This acid then causes cramping and discomfort, thus upsetting you even further and leading to even more acid and churning. So, how to stop this cycle? There are a myriad lifestyle adjustments you could make, many of which we will discuss in the next chapter. For now, however, let's look at a few smaller steps you could easily take when the next bout of anxiety-related cramping or irritated bowel sets in:

- **Drink baking soda:** A deceptively simple kitchen staple, baking soda has more uses than you might have imagined. One of the things it has always been used for is as a digestive aid. Dissolving half a teaspoon of baking soda into a glass of water helps neutralize stomach acids, quickly settling a nervous stomach or working against acid reflux.

- **Use lavender:** Lavender has various well-researched properties that can help settle an upset digestive system and calm the mind (Gladstar, 2008). The scent of lavender itself is tremendously calming, and its essential oil is very safe to use, so adding a drop or two to your pillowcase or even to a scarf or other item of clothing can help ease your mind. Alternatively, make an infusion with dried or fresh lavender leaves, adding a few other calming herbs such as chamomile and lemon balm if you'd like, and drink throughout the day as needed.

- **Avoid caffeine:** Caffeine, especially coffee, is a powerful stimulant, which can set the entire digestive system on a frantic course of action, and irritates the mind as well. If you are prone to feelings of anxiety and related digestive troubles, try cutting down on your coffee intake and observe the difference this makes.

- **Deep breathing:** We discussed breathwork in the previous chapter, but it deserves a recap here. Breathing is an incredibly powerful aid in relaxation and gentle whole-body attunement. Using techniques that focus on lowering the heart rate will also calm the rest of your body, including your gut. I find that even taking two or three minutes to take deep breaths, whenever I find myself becoming flighty or reactive, can make a tremendous difference in the course of my day.

Also, aim to support your digestive system with as wide as possible a variety of herbs and spices. As you now know, your gut flora thrives off variety. Herbs and spices can provide exactly that sense of variety, and they often pack a very strong nutritive punch as well. Making a point to add supportive herbs such as ginger and fennel to your food, or as an infusion, ensures that your belly receives the consistent support that it needs. The next section discusses a few of the most noteworthy medicinal herbs and spices.

Healing Herbs and Spices for Digestive Support

Throughout history, there have been remarkable herbs and spices that have graced the traditions of different cultures… leaving a legacy of digestive wellness. The fact that they have stood the test of time so well, and have been used across so many cultures, speaks of their efficacy.

- **Ginger:** This root has stood the test of time as a reliable ally in soothing digestive discomfort and promoting healthy digestion. Its historical use spans centuries, and across diverse traditional medicine systems, ranging from traditional Chinese medicine to eastern African cultures. Beloved for its calming and warming properties, ginger has been trusted to alleviate a range of digestive issues, such as indigestion, nausea, and bloating. Slow boil slices of ginger root with other beneficial herbs for a delicious tea, or directly add it to your food, as ginger retains its healthy components when cooked.

- **Peppermint:** This herb was recognized by ancient Greek, Roman, and Egyptian cultures for its potential in relieving digestive symptoms and promoting overall digestive wellness. It fares particularly well at easing abdominal pain, reducing bloating, and calming stomach cramps and indigestion. Add some leaves to your salads, or drink it as a cold or warm infusion.

- **Fennel:** This herb is known for its purifying effect, as it stimulates the liver and helps the body detoxify itself. It also improves the appetite, relieves flatulence and bloating, and helps the digestive system retain harmony.

- **Papaya:** This fruit contains so many digestive enzymes that it is even used by some cultures to tenderize meat. Its enzymes significantly help break down proteins, making it a wonderful aid after a heavy or protein-rich meal in particular.

- **Pineapple:** Especially well-loved as a medicinal fruit in South America and Southeast Asia, pineapple is high in bromelain which can help with metabolic functioning and helps resolve indigestion.

- **Turmeric:** This spice truly works for everything. A renowned anti-inflammatory, turmeric also relieves bloating and supports liver functions. It tastes wonderful when added to stews and curries, or consumed as golden milk.

- **Cinnamon:** This spice stimulates the appetite, works as an antifungal, and helps reduce blood sugar. Stir a bit of it into your coffee or tea for a spicy taste, or simply add some to your food where possible.

- **Rosemary:** This is a stimulating herb that also relieves gas and cramping, and helps clear the liver. It tastes wonderful with lamb or chicken, and also works as a wonderful morning stimulant when steeped in some boiling water with lemon juice.

Recipe: Gut-Soothing Ginger and Lemon Infusion

This simple infusion can be made in large batches and refrigerated for consumption throughout the day. It works particularly well against nausea or any stomach irritation, but is equally beneficial to a healthy stomach.

Ingredients:

- 3-inch (or more, if preferred) ginger root, grated or cut into small pieces

- 2 liquid quarts drinking water

- ⅓ cup dried lavender leaves and flowers

- Juice of one lemon

Instructions:

- Put the ginger, lavender and water into a large saucepan and bring it to a boil.

- Once begun boiling, lower the heat and let it simmer for at least 20 minutes, or for as long as one hour, adding more water if too much evaporates.

- Remove from the heat and strain the infusion into a clean container.

- Add the lemon juice, then let cool. Drink throughout the day as desired.

Recipe: Fennel and Papaya Salad

This salad works wonderfully as a digestive aid, both soothing and energizing the entire digestive system. Add yogurt for a delicious breakfast treat, or eat as accompaniment to any meal. The quantities below should serve two people.

Ingredients:

- 1 medium fennel bulb, sliced

- 1 ripe papaya, peeled, seeded, and cut into cubes

- Juice of one lime or lemon

- Fresh mint and basil leaves

- Blueberries, to taste (can also be substituted with another berry of your choice)

- 2 tbsp extra-virgin olive oil

Instructions:

- Combine the papaya, fennel, berries and herbs in a salad bowl.

- In a separate smaller bowl, mix together the olive oil and lime or lemon juice.

- Pour the dressing over the salad, and enjoy!

These two recipes are solitary examples of a wonderful host of flavors and combinations that you could begin to explore in your kitchen. As long as your ingredients are varied and free from pesticides (or, at least, washed well, if organic food isn't available for you), the sky is truly the limit when it comes to experimenting with gut-friendly foods. Play with different flavor possibilities, add different herbs and spices, and over time you'll discover how empowering it feels to have a truly well-supported digestive system and gut biome.

Chapter 6:

Foundation of Strength:

Revitalizing Your Legs and

Feet with Holistic Synergy

Most of us spend a great deal of time thinking about our hair and our faces, about what we eat and whether or not we look and feel good, but one key role player in our health is often overlooked: our feet. We squeeze them into odd shoes, we walk about all day, and we get up in the morning assuming that our legs will carry us wherever we want to go. It is only when we feel a twinge, perhaps after a long day or when an old injury resurfaces, that we really pause to think about our legs and feet. Even then, if it is nothing too serious, we often just hope for the best and carry on. It is only if you have worked as a waiter, or elsewhere in the service industry, that you might understand the importance of your feet, and how they can begin to speak to you when you spend hours standing... day after day.

Our feet may be hardworking and unassuming, but more than almost any other body part, they carry our stories. Surprisingly delicate, especially when you consider the weight they need to carry every day, our feet and legs adapt and change as our lives. For example, did you know that most women's feet become larger during pregnancy, and often do not return to the size they had been before? This is because pregnant women's connective tissues become slightly loose in preparation for giving birth; this affects the arches of their feet, too, where everything moves slightly further apart. By the time the baby is born, the arches of the mother's foot have sunk slightly, making her entire foot a bit longer. This is just one of many ways in which our feet actually make small shifts throughout our lives. Our toes also begin to splay more as we grow older, helping us retain our balance, and our ankles and calves tell the story of every walk and mountain climb we have ever embarked on.

About a quarter of the entire body's bones can be found in the feet. If you think about it, that is an astounding number. There are 206 bones in the human body, and 52 of those are found in the feet alone. On top of that, the feet have hundreds of tendons and ligaments connecting everything together, ensuring mobility and cohesion between each of these bones. The reason for this level of complexity in our feet is quite because their design necessarily needs to be intricate, to allow them to grow, shift, bend, point, and, more importantly, carry us around successfully all our lives. Feet and ankles need to absorb the impact every time we jump or run, while making sure that no other part of the body is injured or impacted too much by our movement.

With more bones and more ligaments, however, comes greater risk of injury. In fact, the ankle is the most commonly injured joint in the body. Apart from tendon, ligament or bone injuries, the lower body can also be prone to swelling and water retention, and can be one of the major places where we experience weakened blood circulation. Tired legs, which is when your feet and legs simply feel heavy and stiff, even when you have not been exercising strenuously, are also quite common. And because the legs and feet support the rest of the body, pain felt elsewhere, such as lower back pain, often originates with the feet. For instance, if you have been walking with a limp, then that imbalance may cause a reference pain higher up, which can only be resolved when the original limp is healed, or, at least, given some relief.

All of this can sound quite terrifying. Most of us are not really experts in foot care, and so we might ask ourselves: How can we, with the limited knowledge that we have, take good care of this important part of our body? The answer is through consistent and loving action, and remembering that our legs and feet form part of the bigger whole, and that what's healthy for the rest of our bodies counts for them, too. Let's now examine some of these actions we can take.

Rest and Recovery: Holistic Techniques for Tired Legs and Feet

In my view, caring for the legs and feet begins with a shift in mindset. Before taking any more tangible action, try to make a point of pondering over your feet for a bit. Think about their importance, and send some gratitude toward them. This small change in focus, when done regularly, brings about a change in how you walk, too, in your posture, in how considerate you are toward your legs and feet. This doesn't mean that you need to coddle them, or stop doing things you love, but imbuing your actions with some gratitude will add some gentleness in your interactions with your own body, ultimately translating into greater wellbeing.

Having said that, here are some tangible things you should also consider doing:

- **Follow the R.I.C.E. method:** RICE stands for "rest-ice-compression-elevation," and it is a well-known technique used to treat injuries. This doesn't mean you should only use it when you are injured or in pain=. I find that applying one or all of these four approaches, whenever I feel even a twinge in my feet, or when I've had a strenuous day, helps to nip injury in the bud immediately. The method is simple: Rest first. Take the weight off your feet. Sit or lie down for a little while. Then apply a pack of frozen peas or an icepack pressed to the part of your legs most prone to injury. This could be the ankle or knee, or even a hamstring (which helps the blood vessels constrict in this area). The body loves contrast, and once the source of cold is removed, blood will rush back to the area with renewed vigor, improving blood circulation, and bringing healing nutrients and oxygen to the area. Compression also works wonders in the form of a knee or ankle brace, or even just a sweater wound tightly around the area. This is important because this compressor holds the affected area safely, making you less prone to odd little movements that may cause an injury to a tired leg. Lastly, elevation helps remove the pressure of blood flowing down toward your legs; thus improving circulation and giving your legs a chance to recover from the everyday toil.

- **Rest your legs up a wall:** This technique has been popular for centuries in many Asian cultures, and with good reason. Lying with your legs up a wall for a few minutes rejuvenates the entire body's circulatory system, helps lymph nodes drain, encourages liver function, gives the back a gentle realignment, and allows your legs to get some rest. If it sounds like an odd exercise, then try combining this with listening to your favorite podcast, or simply doing some breathing exercises. For optimal results, rest a pillow under your hips to make sure your pelvis is higher than your heart.

- **Wear good shoes:** Wearing good shoes doesn't mean wearing only ugly but functional shoes—more and more stylish footwear that do not compromise on comfort is now being made. If your arches, heels or toes hurt regularly, then providing your feet with some more room and support might be the way to go. Alternatively, you could have insoles made specifically for your feet, which can fit into most of the shoes one wears, or buy specialized insoles from a pharmacy. These cushion the feet and support the arches, with the added convenience of being transferable to other shoes when necessary.

- **Notice how you stand:** When we stand, most of us unconsciously shift our weight from foot to foot, lean forward and put too much weight on the toes, or flatten our feet. The next time you are standing—while doing the dishes or cooking, for instance—notice where you put your weight, whether you favor one foot above the other, and whether your feet are a good distance apart. Making minor changes in these areas can radically influence the wellbeing of your feet, and how long you are able to stand overall.

- **Get a massage:** We tend to think of massages as mainly for back problems, but receiving an invigorating leg and foot massage can do wonders for strain injuries and blood circulation. The wonderful thing is that you can also give one to yourself. Try to incorporate foot massages every week, focusing on your arches and the padding of your toes, sending some gratitude to your feet while doing so. Alternatively, try doing a massage swap with a friend or partner.

- **Concentrate on blood circulation:** The body knows best how to naturally heal tiredness or injuries, and it does so through the healing power of oxygenated, nutrient-rich blood. Making sure that the blood supply to your lower extremities is unimpeded is a good way to maintain long-lasting leg health. Do this through dry brushing—the practice of rigorously brushing your legs and feet with a soft-bristled brush—and through alternating hot and cold showers. Stretches and elevation also help with this.

- **Make sure you get enough magnesium:** Magnesium is very important to prevent cramps and ensure suppleness, and so if you are prone to cramping, try to increase your daily magnesium dose. This can be done through regular Epsom salt baths or foot soaks, or through taking a daily magnesium supplement.

Energizing Movement: Exercise for Lower Body Wellbeing

Beyond the small shifts you can begin to incorporate into your way of being in a gentler relationship with your feet, there are also some specific exercises, aimed at the legs and feet, you can begin with. Here is a short list of exercises to start you off:

- **Gentle stretches:** For many of us, the hips are one of the places where we hold the most tension, and even trauma, and similarly, our hamstrings and calves can be significant sites of stress and injury. More and more research is now showing that stretching is not only good for the body, but also heals the mind (van der Kolk, 2014), and incorporating some stretches just before bedtime or during a time of relaxation can do wonders for your general health. Try doing a seated forward fold, with legs slightly bent and body leaning over and above, stretching your arms toward your feet. Another good stretch is bringing your feet together and opening your knees as wide as possible, pushing down on your knees with your elbows to open them even further. Hold the pose for as long as comfortable, and feel how your muscles slowly begin to relax.

- **Toe raises:** This is a tiny exercise, but surprisingly effective in correcting your stance, posture, and any pain in the arches or toes. While standing, move your weight gently to your heels, and try to lift every toe off the ground, splaying them as far apart as possible. If your feet are not particularly flexible, then there may be very little response, but over time, your toes will begin to gain some flexibility, and you'll learn to shift your weight off the front of your feet. Do this exercise while doing anything that requires standing for a while—I particularly like to do it while standing in queues, as it makes the time pass faster and adds a slight humorous edge to the entire experience.

- **Pointing and flexing:** The ankles are often neglected in our exercise routines, and can stiffen quite seriously over time if we do not stretch their range of mobility often enough. To counteract that, simply work some points and flex exercises into your daily routine. You could do this while sitting down and watching a TV show, or any other time when you are sitting and relaxing. Roll your feet in every direction as well, or manually move your ankles around with your hand while supporting your leg with the other arm.

- **Standing calf stretches:** This is similar to a lunge, but more controlled, thus preventing any possible injury. Put one foot against a wall, with the other leg stretched out behind you for balance, and lean forward to touch your hands against the wall as well. Now bend the knee that is facing the wall slowly (your knee should touch the wall as well), while stretching the other leg which is pointing backward. Repeat this a few times for every leg, ensuring that you feel a gentle stretch in the calf that is pointing backward.

- **Calf raises:** These are similarly small exercises that can have a massive impact on your entire leg, particularly on the calf and hamstrings. While standing, shift your weight forward and come onto your tippy toes. Hold that pose for a few seconds, then come down gradually, with as much control as possible. Repeat the exercise a few times, until you feel the stretch in the back and sides of your calves.

- **Low-impact exercise:** While running and participating in sports is never bad for you, it can often lead to repetitive strain injuries, shin splints, or other discomfort across the body. If you find your body asking you to do something gentler for a while, consider doing some low-impact exercise instead. Good examples of this can include swimming, Pilates, walking, and jumping on a rebounder/trampoline. All of these forms of exercise help you move your body and promote flexibility in the legs, without the impact of your entire body weight forcefully hitting your legs and feet.

Soothing Remedies for Happy Feet and Legs

Most of the ingredients that benefit blood circulation and help soothe sore feet have already been featured in Chapter 3. A few notable role players are arnica, turmeric, ginger, lavender and eucalyptus essential oils. Any oil or poultice well-suited to healing back and shoulder pain can be used just as successfully on the legs and feet. On top of that, another ingredient used specifically for tired and swollen feet is the humble potato. Long used in South American and European folk medicine, when applied directly to an affected area, potato reduces inflammation and alleviates swelling, making it perfect for a foot treatment.

Remedy: Potato Foot Mask for Aching Feet

This mask is easy to make and wonderfully effective for any swelling or skin irritation. Apply it to your feet after a long day, or simply when you need some pampering.

Ingredients:

- 1 medium-sized potato, boiled and mashed

- 1 tbsp coconut oil

- 1 tbsp honey

- 2-3 drops essential oil of your choice

Instructions:

- Mix all the ingredients nicely in a bowl, until a smooth paste is formed.

- Layer the paste evenly on clean feet, either covering your feet entirely or focusing on the painful areas.

- Leave the mask on for about 15 minutes, or until it starts to dry.

- Rinse off with lukewarm water, pat your feet dry, and apply a gentle moisturizer.

Recipe: Turmeric and Ginger Foot Soak

Ingredients:

- 1 tbsp turmeric powder
- 1 tbsp grated ginger
- 2 tbsp Epsom salt
- Warm water

Instructions:

Stir the Epsom salt into water until it has dissolved, and then add ginger and turmeric; stir again. Soak your feet in the water for about 20 minutes, massaging them occasionally to enhance blood circulation.

Chapter 7:

The Holistic Nexus:

Cultivating Synergistic

Wellbeing for Your Body, Mind,

and Spirit

When talking about holistic wellness, it is important to keep in mind more than just the body. After all, the word "holistic" implies "whole." To be well in the truest sense of the word, we need to bring our bodies, minds, and spirits into unity: to be whole on more than just a physical level. As we know by now, when it comes to wellness, everything has an impact on everything else. What we eat affects our entire body, but it also affects the mind, through the mind-gut connection. Similarly, the heart is affected by our thoughts and emotions. This works both ways: We can nourish the mind and spirit by taking care of the body, but we can also nourish the body by taking care of the less tangible aspects of ourselves. Now that we have discussed most of the physical aspects of wellbeing, it is time we took a closer look at the mind-body-spirit nexus.

To do that, we need to be clear on what we mean by the words "mind" and "spirit." What is *spirit?* The concept has been with us since ancient times, and can be found in most cultures' written texts. It changes meaning slightly from age to age, depending on a culture's transforming world views, but it always boils down to the same idea: the heart and energy inside every person, the part of us that is moved by beauty and longs for connection and meaning. You could perhaps view this as a person's inner fire; as the beautiful energy that makes every person unique. Although some people attach their own spiritual worldviews to the concept, and are definitely free to do so, there is no inherently religious link to the word "spirit." It simply means each of our vibrant, inner selves.

Mind is more closely linked to the brain, and particularly to thoughts and emotions. Like spirit, this concept has been with us since the beginning of time. In the context of this book, we'll use it to describe our cognitive decision-making skills, the way we make sense of the world, our likes and dislikes, and how we structure our lives. Can you feel that this is somewhat different from "spirit"? These overlap, of course, just like "body" and "mind" overlap, since all three concepts are interconnected and deeply affect each other. This is good news, since taking care of one aspect means taking care of all, and there is no set starting point. To nourish your entire being, simply begin from where you are, acknowledging that you are a complex being with many interdependent needs. Since we have spent much time focusing on the body already, and the next chapter deals more closely with the mind, let's look at some of the ways that can lead to whole-body health via nourishing the spirit.

Building Meaning Into Daily Life

In my understanding of it, nourishing the spirit simply means to imbue our daily lives with meaning. Psychotherapist and Holocaust survivor Viktor Frankl wrote in his book, *Man's Search for Meaning* (1946), that humans are capable of dealing with great hardships, as long as they have a reason to do so, and can hold onto something that they believe in. Think of hardships you have overcome: Did you have a goal at the end of your suffering which helped you get through it? We are motivated to study for exams because we know that the end results will be worth it; we tirelessly care for our children because we love them and believe in their future; we work on our relationships because we long for connection and intimacy. We are capable of doing surprisingly difficult things every day, simply because we know those things to be worth it.

The first step toward cultivating meaning in our lives is thus to identify what is important to us. In other words, to find your values. Once you have done that, it becomes easier to build your life around these values, increasingly filling your days with things that are meaningful. Here are a few questions you could ask yourself to identify what's most important to you:

- Looking at your life right now: What in it gives you a deep, warm sense of love or enjoyment? If you answer "my children" or "my work,", try to dig a bit deeper. What is it about your children that gives you this sense of warmth and love? Is it their ability to laugh and be spontaneous, their innocence, the hope they represent, the fact that they love you back? At work, is it the thrill of doing something well, the connection with your colleagues, the comfort of the routine, or the fact that your job makes a difference in the world? Write down all the answers that come to you. These are all pointing you toward where you find true meaning.

- Which qualities do you value the most in yourself and other people? Write down all the words that come to you—these point you to your principles.

- What kind of life do you dream of having? Is it full of nature, or beautiful art, or animals, or stimulating work? Do you imagine it as busy and energizing, or gentle and slow? Write down all the words that come to you, as all of them point you toward your values.

Rediscovering Balance: Nurturing the Body-Mind-Spirit Connection

Once you have a better understanding of your values and what motivates you, you can begin to consciously point your life in the direction of the things that excite you. Since the mind, body, and spirit are so intricately linked, the best way to nourish this connection is by matching your values with some tangible actions that involve both your mind and body. Let's take a look at some of the ways you could begin to do this:

- **Connect to nature:** Research has frequently shown that humans do better when they regularly engage with nature (Delagran, 2011; Kaplan, 1995). How you do so depend on your unique values and circumstances, however. If you value quiet and restfulness, then consider finding a park or isolated place in nature where you can go to unwind. If you like engaging in activities, then you could start a herb garden, or participate in nature hikes. Engaging with nature can also be combined with community activities, such as joining a community garden, joining a nature interest group or NGO, or simply involving friends in your nature walks.

- **Connect with animals:** This forms part of the previous point, since animals are part of nature (as are we). You might not consider yourself an animal lover, and you don't need to volunteer at your local animal shelter to connect with animals. Sometimes, simply noticing your environment is all it takes. Start paying attention to the morning birdsong outside your window, get curious about the varied animal life populating your town or city, or simply watch an animal documentary every now and again. Becoming aware of the various life forms around us has shown to increase our sense of meaning and offer us a sense of belonging—realizing that we humans are not alone on this planet also helps us take more conscious responsibility for our environment and tread with more awareness.

- **Cultivate a gratitude practice:** An increasing amount of science is now pointing us toward the fact that cultivating gratitude has a tremendous impact on both physical and emotional health (Allen, 2018). To tap into these benefits, try starting a small gratitude practice. This could be as simple as thinking about some things you are grateful for every morning, while enjoying your favorite morning drink. You could also start keeping a gratitude journal, or even involve a loved one by telling each other about the things you are grateful for.

- **Build community:** Humans are social beings, and whether you consider yourself an intro- or extrovert, you are no exception to this. We fare better when we feel a sense of belonging, and are surrounded by people who mean something to us. So, nurture your relationships, both your most intimate ones and those further afield. This means making a point to maintain your closest relationships, learning to communicate well, learning to make boundaries so that you don't become depleted in the service of others, and finding your own personal balance between social and solo activities. It can also mean finding a cause you believe in and becoming active toward furthering it—you can do so by joining a conversation group, volunteering with some friends, becoming involved in a local civil society group, or taking up a meaningful hobby.

- **Turn your routines into rituals:** We all have habits and routines, though we might not always be aware of them. Perhaps, you get up at roughly the same time every morning, drink a cup of coffee, then jump in the shower, and head off to work. Perhaps, you find yourself taking a breather at work at roughly the same time every day, or perhaps you are quite attached to the TV show you and your partner watch every evening after supper. These are all routines, and by simply adding a bit more awareness of those activities, you can turn them into meaningful rituals, imbuing them with a sense of specialness and presence. For example, if you have coffee every morning, then try to do this more mindfully, savoring every sip, perhaps while sitting outside and looking at the brightening day. If you and your partner watch the same show every evening, try to take a moment to smile and reconnect with each other before sinking into the couch, acknowledging the sweetness of your shared "ritual." The more we fill our days with tiny conscious moments, the more meaning begins to permeate our lives.

Body-Based Practices for Enhancing Inner Harmony

Having discussed some of the larger themes and practices that nourish the connection between our bodies and inner beings, let's now take a look at some particular body-based strategies which help our entire selves come into harmony. You'll see that we have discussed or mentioned many of these already—and this is because what's good for the body is good for the spirit, and vice versa.

- **Breathing:** We have been speaking about the power of breathing throughout this book. On top of the health benefits it offers, keep in mind that this is also one of the simplest, yet potent, ways of bringing the body and spirit into harmony. Even just a few minutes of mindful breathing per day may produce tremendous benefits.

- **Stretching:** This one has also been discussed already, so it is sufficient to say that bringing some stretches into your daily life is an effective way of shedding some stress and getting in touch with parts of your body you might normally not pay much attention to. Add some stretches to your evening routine, or stretch after an hour or two's work, and see the difference it starts to make.

- **Dance or freeform movement:** This can take on various forms, depending on your personality, but any form of dancing or free movement, especially to music, has repeatedly been shown to release endorphins and other feel-good hormones, and help us get in touch with our bodies in a more intuitive way. If the thought of dancing makes you feel shy, then start small: Sway back and forth to music in your kitchen, where no one can see you, or simply add music to other daily forms of exercises, bringing some spontaneity into your movements. Alternatively, signing up for a dancing class, whether ballroom, Latin, or any other form of your choice/interest, can provide some structure within which you may become more used to moving your body in innovative ways.

- **Mind-body practices:** These include all kinds of exercises aimed at bringing together movement, breathing, and body awareness, and can include martial arts and Pilates. These practices are particularly good at improving your proprioceptive—awareness of your own body in space, and helping you become gently aware of your reflexive patterns, such as how you may tend to breathe more shallowly during a stressful time.

- **Swimming:** Because our bodies are lighter in water, we are immediately plunged into a more freeing experience through swimming than we can possibly experience elsewhere. Swimming doesn't need to entail doing many laps in a large swimming pool, although you could certainly do that if you'd like. Taking a dip in a lake every now and again, or splashing about with your kids at a local pool can be just as beneficial.

- **Mindful walking:** Incorporate mindful breathing into your next walk, and try to pay attention to your environment: notice the trees, the streets you walk through, your breathing, and the sensation of walking itself. You'll soon find yourself tapping into surprising depths of joy and meaning through this simple act.

Ingredients That Feed Your Soul

Plants do not just nourish the body; they also nourish the soul, and in more ways than one. Many herbs, spices, and plant extracts contain ingredients that help lift the spirits, clear the mind, and soothe the heart. On top of that, the essential oils of various sweet-smelling plants have been used for centuries in what is today known as aromatherapy, a well-researched—and easily accessible—form of therapeutic treatment. Below are some of the most noteworthy aromatherapy and consumable ingredients to feed your soul:

- **Ashwagandha:** An ancient healing herb, ashwagandha is used for a wide variety of purposes: from helping the body withstand stress and improving sleep quality to retaining vitality and vigor.

- **Ginseng:** This root has been used for a very long time in traditional Chinese medicine, and quickly became popular in the western world with the rise of globalization. It helps boost both physical and mental energy.

- **Rosemary:** An energizing, fragrant herb, rosemary enhances concentration and also helps provide mental and emotional clarity.

- **Essential oils:** Chamomile, lavender, bergamot, ylang-ylang and myrrh, these oils, in particular, have a calming or gently stimulating effect on the mood, but you could use any other essential oils you like. Add a few drops to your bath, or use them in a diffuser to permeate your home with their scent.

Recipe: *Ashwagandha Elixir*

This fragrant drink can also be combined with turmeric to make a soul-nourishing golden milk, or you could add other spices according to your own taste.

Ingredients:

- 1 tsp ashwagandha powder
- 1 cup milk or milk substitute
- 1 tsp honey
- ½ tsp ground cinnamon

Instructions:

- Heat the milk in a saucepan, taking care not to let it boil.
- Remove the milk from the heat and stir in the rest of the ingredients, making sure that they have blended well into the milk.
- Sip the elixir slowly for maximum enjoyment—this drink is meant to be savored.

Chapter 8:

Inner Radiance: Unlocking the Synergy of Holistic Healing for Your Mind

In the previous chapter, we delved into the importance of approaching wellness from more than just a physical standpoint. The mind and spirit are inextricably connected to the body, and therefore taking care of one's emotional wellbeing matters just as much as eating well or having a healthy beauty routine does. In particular, we looked at some of the ways in which emotional wellbeing may be cultivated, through creating meaning for ourselves and connecting with the living world. From that spiritual perspective, we now move to a focus on the mind: that is looking at how we may improve our memory, focus, and ability to complete tasks. The mind is also connected to the brain, which can be kept healthy in many tangible ways—this is also something we'll investigate in the following pages.

Holistic Approaches to Cultivating Mental Wellbeing

The human brain is an incredible organ, and we have just recently really begun to really understand it—much remains to be learned. What we do know is that the brain weighs only about 2% of our entire body mass, yet consumes about 20% of our metabolic energy, making it the most fuel-intensive part of our entire body (Mergenthaler, 2013). Research has also shown that the brain is more plastic than we had imagined before (van der Kolk, 2014). This means that new neural connections and pathways can be formed throughout our lives, allowing us to learn more new skills and develop new habits into old age. If you have been suffering from brain fog or poor concentration, this doesn't have to be your lot forever. There are various things you can do to significantly improve your brain functioning, and many of these have actually already been discussed in this book. For example, consuming foods high in polyphenols and flavonoids, which we discussed in several previous chapters, is a great option to enhance brain functioning. These foods include leafy green vegetables, broccoli, pumpkin seeds, berries, and dark chocolate. Regular exercise is equally good for the brain, particularly if you engage in forms of exercise that stimulate the mind—mindful walking and proprioception exercises are good examples of this. Apart from the holistic wellness ideas we have discussed so far, here are a few more you could try bringing into your life, which are sure to energize and train your mind:

- **Mental stimulation:** To successfully move through our days, most of us fall into habits: both habits of action and mental habits. This includes our automatic morning routines, the road we take to work, the automated way we might set about cleaning the house, picking the kids up from school, walking the dog, and doing a host of other routine tasks. This is not a bad thing—habits help us entrench beneficial behaviors. However, the mind needs regular stimulation, in the form of newness and renewed mindfulness. One way of doing this is to occasionally change up your routine— take a different route to work every now and then, go somewhere by using a map instead of the GPS, or switch up your exercise routine. Exposing ourselves to new information is also an excellent way of stimulating the mind: Listen to podcasts about interesting topics, read a few pages from a book rather than watching TV, try to learn a new language. There are now even dozens of smartphone apps meant to stimulate the mind with a variety of puzzles and brainteasers, many of which have been scientifically researched and proven to improve brain plasticity.

- **Engage in hobbies:** This links up with our previous point—hobbies are an excellent way to keep the brain engaged and provide it with new things to think about. If you don't think you have the time for hobbies, then listen to podcasts or eBooks about a topic that interests you. Alternatively, you could combine a hobby with a social activity, by inviting friends to come along to pottery class or whichever other activity you'd like to start up. Your hobby could be very small—learning the names of the trees along your daily walk, cultivating a few perennial herbs on your windowsill—but tiny as it may be, as long as it grabs your attention and retains it, your brain is being exercised in a new avenue which is hugely beneficial for its continued vigor.

- **Quality sleeping:** Most of us need between 7.5 and 8.5 hours of sleep a day, and it is important that we do get a good quality slumber. Try to protect your sleep at all costs. If you tend to struggle with insomnia or bad quality of sleep, focus on cultivating good sleep hygiene: Avoiding screens after 8 PM, refraining from drinking caffeine after a certain time, eating supper early enough that digestion and sleeping time don't coincide, and ensuring that your room is dark enough for good sleep can be good starting points. Slowly you'll begin to notice yourself sleeping better and better, and the effects on the rest of your life will immediately become apparent.

- **Stress management:** Most of us live lives that are overwhelmingly driven by stress and the resulting stress hormones, cortisol and adrenaline. While both hormones can be good in the short run, when their levels constantly remain high, they begin to affect our physical health as well as the health of our minds. If you find yourself frequently feeling overwhelmed/irritated/tired at the end of your tether, then it is probably time to reshuffle some aspects of your life. This may feel impossible to do at first—it may feel as if everything in your life is clamoring for attention, and nothing can easily be put aside. If that is the case, then you may need to establish stronger boundaries, ruthlessly prioritize certain tasks above others, and perhaps let certain activities go (though not the ones that give you joy). Enlist the help of a loved one to do this, or get an accountability partner to help you cut down on sources of stress in your life. Allow yourself to imagine a life filled with peace—it is feasible, and you totally deserve to have that life.

- **Limit screen time:** Most of us spend a ridiculous amount of time staring at our screens, alert to every notification that flashes across, never far away from the endless array of emails and social media willing to distract us from our lives. In my case, it took me a solitary seven-day retreat to realize how addicted I had become to my phone. There I was, surrounded by nature and silence, yet every few minutes I would reflexively pick up my phone to see whether any new messages had come in. Once I realized this, I made the conscious choice to detox myself from my phone—and it took some doing. Our brains have now been trained to seek our phones as a constant source of entertainment and quick dopamine hits. But the brain is plastic, which means that it can be trained to find joy elsewhere. To do this, set aside a few hours of screen-free time every day, or even try to keep your phone on airplane mode for a predetermined period of time. Soon the noise outside and even inside your mind will quieten, and beauty will be given a renewed chance to seep in.

Nutrition to Enhance Cognitive Function

We have already taken a brief look at some of the foods that help support optimal brain functioning, but there are also particular herbs, minerals, and plant extracts that can play a hugely beneficial role in brain health. Many of these ingredients are called adaptogens, which are a class of plants and fungi renowned for their ability to support the body through times of stress and enhance mental clarity. Here are the most significant supplements and adaptogens you should consider adding to your pantry:

- **Sage:** This beautiful pale green herb is known for its cognition enhancing properties. It is also believed to counteract age-related mental decline. Use the herb dried or fresh in food, steep it in boiling water, or add a few drops of its essential oil to your bath.

- **Peppermint:** This herb has long been used by various cultures to help improve mental clarity and focus. It tastes delicious in salads and can be added to tea—or you could simply chew a leaf every now and then, freshening your breath and your mental clarity at the same time.

- **Lemon balm:** This herb was particularly popular in various European healing traditions. It contains various compounds that help with relaxation, deep sleep, and renewed concentration. It is related to the mint family, and can be consumed in the same ways as peppermint.

- **Holy basil:** This unassuming and fragrant herb doesn't only spruce up a pasta sauce or salads; it is also widely known for its calming effects, and for its memory-enhancing results.

- **Gotu kola:** A sweet-looking plant that grows abundantly almost anywhere, and can often be picked on nature walks or even on sidewalks, gotu kola is a powerful neuroprotective agent and can significantly improve memory and brain function. Whenever I see gotu kola growing anywhere, I make a point to pick a few leaves and eat it raw or add it to my next salad plate—this plant is potent enough that a few leaves here and there can make a huge difference.

- **Ginkgo biloba:** The gingko biloba tree is one of the oldest trees known to mankind. It is native to Japan and extremely renowned for its healing properties. Buy ginkgo biloba extract from any pharmacy and drink it as a regular supplement for optimal benefits.

- **Lion's mane mushroom:** Extracts from this mushroom are showing tremendous effects on the production of new cell growth, meaning that lion's mane may help with brain plasticity and improve learning ability. It is often used to counteract cognitive decline in aging people.

- **Bacopa monnieri:** Also known as water hyssop, this wetland herb has been found to enhance memory, learning, and cognitive performance.

- **Rhodiola rosea:** This flowering plant, native to the northernmost parts of the Earth, is a well-known adaptogen, known for its ability to reduce fatigue and stress levels and improving attention span. You can buy the extract at any pharmacy.

- **Reishi mushroom:** An astoundingly multi-purpose mushroom, reishi helps with neuroplasticity and brain recovery, on top of being tremendously beneficial for wound healing and general health.

Recipe: Brain-Boosting Ginkgo Biloba Smoothie

This smoothie combines the nutritious power of foods high in flavonoids and antioxidants, such as bananas and berries, with the brain-boosting effects of ginkgo biloba. Add some reishi powder for extra benefits, or change up the fruits according to your taste.

Ingredients:

- 1 tsp ginkgo biloba powder
- 1 cup yogurt, or any dairy substitute
- ½ cup blueberries, fresh or frozen
- 1 banana
- 1 tbsp nut butter

Instructions:

Combine all the ingredients into a blender and mix well. The recipe is enough for two servings, so consider sharing it with someone.

Many of the ingredients discussed in the previous chapter are also very beneficial for brain health—in fact, the vast majority of the ingredients discussed throughout this book equally benefit the brain. So, make the ideas, listed here and in the other chapters, your own—chopping and changing as you deem fit. Remember, the body is an integrated system, which means you don't have to consume a different supplement for every body part. Instead, using variations of a few trusted recipes, such as the smoothie above, will be sure to benefit your entire system.

Chapter 9:

Inner Symphony: Holistic Support for Optimal Organ Harmony and Balance

The human body is nothing short of miraculous. The number of processes that take place within the body every hour is breathtaking—breathing, circulation, digestion, hormone release, metabolism, waste elimination, temperature regulation, nerve signaling, and cell regeneration, among others. Now ask yourself: How many of these processes are you even aware of? Probably very few, and you might have conscious control over even fewer of these. This is because most of these actions are controlled by the autonomic nervous system, which is responsible for all the unconscious and reflexive actions our bodies are consistently taking. Imagine the autonomic nervous system as a night watchman, constantly monitoring dozens of cameras and overseeing what happens where, allowing you to rest while all this happens. It would be absolutely impossible for us to split our conscious attention into all these various tasks—remembering to tell the heart to beat and the gut to digest would be akin to a full-time job, let alone the hundreds of other interconnected tasks that take place at the same time, too.

Just because we are not aware of, or have complete, conscious control over all our autonomic functions, doesn't mean that we have no influence over what happens within our bodies. We absolutely can and do have an impact on the functioning of our various organs, and on how well they work together. This should not be a scary thought, but rather an empowering one—you are not at the mercy of an automated system. Your thoughts, habits, and conscious behaviors can positively influence the functioning of your entire system.

The first step toward supporting the functioning of all your internal organs is to inform yourself about them. Having an awareness of the complexity and sophistication of the bodily systems helps you treat your body with a renewed appreciation. Most of us learn very little about our bodies at school—a few perfunctory biology modules, at best—which, if you think about it, is rather odd, since we spend so much time analyzing poetry and memorizing geometric theorems. Fortunately, that can be corrected: We can learn and become acquainted with our bodies, and learn how to take responsibility for this miraculous system. This book is one step in that direction, and this chapter in particular aims to empower you with knowledge about how your internal organs work as a series of perfectly interwoven systems.

The Internal Organs

So far, we have investigated the function and care of quite a few of the organs: the skin, the heart, the digestive system (comprising more than one organ), and the brain. Various other organs remain, and for the purposes of this book we'll discuss four more here: pancreas, liver, kidneys, and lungs. All of these organs fulfill vital functions, but they are often shrouded in some mystery for us. Let's demystify them together.

The Liver

The liver is the second largest organ in the human body (the first being the skin), and is involved in various vital functions. Did you know that the liver can regrow itself even when as much as 90% has been removed? (Reynolds, 2021). This wonderful organ can withstand more than most other parts of our bodies, particularly because it is responsible for detoxifying the body. It filters toxins and waste products from the bloodstream, metabolizes nutrients, stores glucose, and helps regulate blood sugar. It also plays a key role in strengthening the immune system through synthesizing proteins, transporting nutrients to different parts of the body, and storing vitamins and minerals. Because the liver is involved in so many filtering and detoxifying processes, it is exposed to all the toxins that enter the body, and even though it is largely able to regenerate itself, it can be severely damaged by alcohol, strong medication, microplastics, and other environmental toxins. Supporting the liver, therefore, means helping it detoxify itself, giving it the occasional break from filtering harmful substances by eating only pure, simple foods and herbs for a while that are specialized at supporting liver functions. We'll discuss all of these in later sections of this chapter.

The Kidneys

Two bean-shaped organs located near the lower back, the kidneys have the important role of filtering waste and excess water by producing urine. By doing this, they also regulate the fluid balance in the body, maintain the body's acid-base balance, and regulate blood pressure by managing the balance of electrolyte, water, and hormones that affect how blood vessels constrict and dilate. To me, kidneys are an excellent example of how bodily processes interact with and affect each other—a process as seemingly simple as filtering toxins from the blood impacts on blood pressure, hormone levels, hydration, and pH in the entire body. Because the kidneys, like the liver, filter toxins, they need particular care and support to remain healthy throughout one's life. Kidney care is, therefore, focused on decreasing intake of toxins, consuming beneficial electrolytes, and drinking ample water. We'll discuss further specific steps later in this chapter.

The Lungs

In a way, the lungs are the body's main point of contact with the outside world. Even more than the digestive system, they take in and process a life-giving resource from outside the body—in this case, oxygen, which is then distributed throughout the bloodstream with the help of the heart. Because the lungs also control carbon dioxide levels in the body, they play a role in acid-base balancing, too, along with the kidneys; on top of that, they also act as one of the body's primary defense mechanisms, which they perform by trapping incoming pathogens and foreign substances. While the liver and kidneys are responsible for expelling toxins, the lungs keep them out of the body in the first place. Similar to the previous two organs, then, it is very important that the lungs are supported in their function as detoxifiers and defenders of the body.

The Pancreas

A much lesser-appreciated organ, the pancreas is a glandular organ, and so, to some degree, it actually forms part of the endocrine system. This means that it produces hormones such as insulin that help regulate blood sugar levels, and thus help the body process food. It also has an exocrine function, which means that it produces digestive enzymes, thus supporting the small intestine in its digestive functions. Support for the pancreas is focused on controlling blood sugar levels which allows it to function with greater ease.

Discussions about the pancreas remain incomplete without understanding the endocrine system. This system is made up of various glands, each of which counts as its own organ. These glands, situated all across the body and varying in size, are responsible for most of the body's hormonal production, acting as chemical messengers, regulating aspects of metabolism, reproduction, and growth and development. It can be harder to get a handle on this system than other organs because it is so complex and interconnected, and works in close co-operation with the nervous system. However, this doesn't mean that caring for the endocrine system needs to remain a mystery— support for this system focuses on ensuring that the body's needs are met so that it can function optimally.

Strengthening Vital Organs: A Holistic Approach

Now that we have some grasp on most of the body's organs and how they work together, let's investigate how best to take care of them. First of all, here are some general steps that will benefit all of your organs:

- **Stay hydrated:** The body is made up of 55-60% water, which means that staying hydrated is absolutely essential for every cell in our bodies. Water also plays a key role in almost all our autonomous functions, with the kidneys and endocrine system, in particular, needing proper hydration. Depending on the size of your body, you should try to drink about 60 fluid ounces (two liters) of water every day. If you feel that your kidneys need extra support, for example, after drinking some alcohol or when you have been ill, then consider adding some electrolytes to your water as well, such as Himalayan salt, a pinch of cream of tartar, and Epsom salts.

- **Avoid refined sugars and simple carbs where possible:** One of the foundations of a holistic health approach is to avoid becoming fixated on "bad foods." This means that no food should be demonized, not even highly processed foods and sugar, since this causes an imbalanced and fearful approach. Having said that, the body really thrives off complex, fibrous carbohydrates, rather than simple sugars. The pancreas, in particular, has a much easier time regulating blood sugar levels when refined sugar doesn't throw it off kilter too often, and the gut and liver, too, need nutrient-rich foods.

- **Move:** Try to shift your focus from "exercise every day"—which feels like a command and can become another source of stress—to "regularly move your body" instead. Movement can come in many guises: climbing the stairs, gardening, stretching, walking the dog, dancing in your kitchen, or splashing in the pool with the kids. Exercise is important to every organ in the body, but this doesn't mean that you need to stick to a rigid exercise routine. Rather, make movement work for you, and revel in the knowledge that your body is thanking you.

- **Sleep:** This is another lifestyle factor that can become a source of stress for many of us. There is nothing worse than lying wide awake, watching the time pass, and becoming more and more anxious as the night ticks away. Yes, sleep is important, especially to the endocrine system and the brain, but allow yourself to relax around this issue as well. Practice good sleep hygiene, or work naps into your day if you struggle at night. If nothing works, then spend your bedtime hours systematically relaxing your body and regulating your breathing. Often, all it takes for sleep to come is to stop obsessing over its absence.

- **Be judicious with alcohol and other substances:** This doesn't mean you should never drink alcohol—in fact, some studies show that a small amount of red wine can be beneficial for the body (Buettner, 2010). However, when you do decide to drink alcohol, try to support your body even more than usual in other ways: Drink water, sleep enough, and eat a healthy meal the next day. In particular, make a point of supporting the liver by consuming herbs and foods that help it recover.

Herbs and Foods for Organ Health

Most of the foods that are particularly good for organ health have already been mentioned in this book, proving again that with a holistic system, like the body, what's good for one part is good for the whole. To recap what these foods are: For optimal health, eat leafy greens, healthy fats, berries and other colorful foods high in flavonoids, nuts and seeds, and cruciferous vegetables such as broccoli and cabbage. On top of that, here are some foods and herbs that particularly benefit specific organs—consume these when you'd like to specifically support the organ in question.

- **Garlic:** Good for the entire body, garlic specifically helps activate liver enzymes, thus helping it eliminate toxins. Some of its compounds also help reduce the risk of kidney disease.

- **Turmeric:** The unquestioned superstar in this book, the anti-inflammatory compounds in turmeric support the liver and heart functioning.

- **Green tea:** The antioxidants in green tea help protect the liver and lungs from damage.

- **Olive oil:** The anti-inflammatory components in olive oil support the kidneys particularly well.

- **Tomatoes:** Tomatoes contain an antioxidant called lycopene, which helps protect the lungs against damage.

- **Ginger:** This powerful herb not only soothes the entire digestive system, but also supports the liver in its detoxifying functions, and benefits lung health, too.

- **Milk thistle:** This herb supports liver health and helps promote detoxification.

- **Dandelion:** This plant helps promote the flow of bile, thus supporting the liver in its processes, while also promoting good kidney functioning. Other bitter herbs, such as arugula, mustard greens and bitter lettuce, are all hugely beneficial to the liver, too.

- **Cranberry:** This berry contains compounds that prevent harmful bacteria from infecting the urinary tract, thus supporting the kidneys and the entire detoxifying system.

- **Oil of oregano:** The essential oil of oregano is a tremendously powerful antimicrobial and antioxidant. Use it topically against infections or for an immune system boost—its beneficial compounds will be absorbed by the skin and reach the necessary organs, particularly the liver and kidneys. Small doses can even be dropped into the ears (for ear infection) or taken orally, as long as this is done sparingly and with caution.

Supporting Detoxification and Cleansing

You may have heard that detoxes and cleanses are not really necessary, since the liver and kidneys detox themselves—that's what they are there for, after all. It is indeed true that many detox fads are entirely unnecessary and can even sometimes be dangerous. The liver and kidneys do a good job in detoxing the entire body. However, they do need some help sometimes. Particularly when you have been ill, sleeping badly, or ingesting more toxins than usual, the liver can become sluggish and exhausted, and your kidneys less efficient. Tired kidneys can lead to bladder and kidney infections, or dehydration and swelling, while a sluggish liver can become diseased over time. Fortunately, there are some simple things you can do to support your body in its detoxifying functions. Improved blood circulation means improved cleansing, so dry brushing your skin, lying with your legs up a wall, and jumping on a rebounder all help the liver better fulfill its functions. Bitter herbs and tonics also support your detoxifying organs. If you feel truly sick and stagnant, then eating fewer fatty foods for a few days, or even going on a water fast for a while, can give the liver a much-needed break from the work it normally needs to do, thus allowing it to revive itself.

Recipe: Detoxifying Dandelion Tea

Ingredients:

- 2 tbsp dried dandelion leaves or root
- 1 and a ½ cup hot water
- A few whole cloves
- 1 tsp lemon juice

Instructions

Steep the dried dandelion and cloves in hot water for 15 minutes, then strain the infusion into a clean container. Add the lemon juice and enjoy hot or cold.

Chapter 10:

Synergistic Nutrition: Fueling Your Body and Mind

In our quest for holistic health, incorporating nutrient-dense foods into our diet is a powerful way to fuel our bodies and promote overall wellbeing. Food has featured prominently in every chapter of this book, more because it is one of the primary ways we can support our bodies from top to toe. You have also seen certain foods mentioned again and again, such as healthy fats, colorful vegetables, dark leafy greens, and high-quality protein. By now, you probably have a good understanding of what a healthy diet entails; in this chapter we'll cement that understanding, focusing on practical ways to build good nourishment into our daily lives. This is done by prioritizing a balanced meal plan, embracing a variety of foods, exploring superfoods, and considering each unique body's nutritional and hormonal needs. By following a gentle, non-prescriptive approach, focusing on enjoying a variety of beautiful and healthy foods, we can truly nourish ourselves from within.

Creating a Balanced Plate: The Well-Rounded Approach

At the heart of a nutrient-dense diet lies the concept of a balanced meal. The body needs the three macronutrients on a regular basis: fat, protein, and carbohydrates. All foods that we consume are made largely of these macronutrients, with various micronutrients (vitamins and minerals) being present in most foods, too. As a rule of thumb, a balanced meal entails roughly 40% carbohydrates, 40% protein, and 20% fats. In terms of serving size, an approach that helps me keep track of how much to eat is the "fist rule", which is based on the size of your own fist: Per meal, eat roughly one fist of carbs, one fist of proteins, and half a fist of fats.

However, not all proteins, carbs, or fats are created equally—for instance, while half a sweet potato and three slices of white bread might both be roughly the size of your fist, they do not pack nearly similar nutritional punches. It is therefore important to be conscious of the quality of your food, too. Here are a few things to keep in mind when planning your meals:

- Choose whole-grain over refined grains wherever possible. Grains can be a nutritious source of carbs, but only when they have not been too refined. Refined carbs contain far less fiber, and are made up of simple carbs rather than complex carbs. The body breaks down simple carbs into sugars in no time, spiking the blood sugar in the process and putting more strain on the liver and pancreas, while complex carbs ensure a more gradual release of energy. Choose whole-wheat bread and pasta, and alternate these two choices with brown rice, buckwheat, and quinoa whenever possible.

- Starchy vegetables are also a good source of carbs. You don't need to rely only on grains for your daily intake of carbs—in fact, starchy vegetables make for excellent alternatives to pasta and bread. Experiment with incorporating sweet potatoes, potatoes, carrots, beets, and squashes into your diet, especially if you can buy them organically grown. Not only do these provide slow-release carbs, but their starch contents also feed the good bacteria in your gut, ensuring a healthy microbiome.

- Leafy greens and other vegetables contain both protein and carbs. When calculating how many proteins and carbs to eat, don't forget that most vegetables contain a bit of both. Even seemingly flimsy leafy greens such as lettuce, spinach, and kale can significantly contribute to your daily carb needs. I find that adding extra cauliflower and broccoli to my plate, for instance, decreases my need to eat a lot of rice or pasta. Similarly, some vegetables can be quite high in protein—mung bean and alfalfa sprouts, spinach, mustard greens, and asparagus can all form part of your daily protein intake.

- Protein doesn't have to equal meat. This relates to what we have just discussed—protein can come in many forms, including plant-based forms. If you eat meat, then that can indeed be a healthy source of protein for you, as long as the animal it came from was grass-fed or caught from the wild, but there are other options, too. Eggs are wonderful sources of protein, and if you are a vegan, then legumes and tofu can also provide you with your daily dose of protein.

- For daily fats, use dressings and toppings. Many foods naturally contain some fat, including dairy and most other animal products. On top of that, we often fry food in oil (hopefully using a healthy oil such as coconut or MCT oil). That often is not enough to fulfill our daily fat requirements, however. To solve that, make your own salad dressings using olive or flaxseed oil, drizzle some sesame oil over your stir-fry, add guacamole as a side dish or avocado as a topping, add nut butters to your food, and sprinkle grilled nuts and seeds over your salads.

- Switch things up: As we discussed in the chapter on gut health, the gut microbiome thrives on diversity. While most of us have a few food staples we rely on, a few favorite dishes we like to cook, it's also important that we challenge ourselves with new foods and new tastes. Doing this ensures that we receive all the micronutrients we need in our diets, and, of course, that we broaden our culinary horizons. The more interesting foods you add to your diet, the more you will open yourself to the fun of food—and having fun is central to maintaining a sustainable, healthy diet. Add variety to your diet by adding various fresh herbs and even some medicinal plants to your salads—dandelion, yarrow, feverfew, holy basil, radish greens, gotu kola, among others. Keep a few healthy oils in your food closet and alternate between them. Occasionally try eating kohlrabi instead of cabbage, rainbow trout instead of salmon, or buckwheat instead of couscous. Add spices such as cloves, cumin, and allspice to your tea. Experiment with fermented foods, and make dishes from a cuisine you are not very familiar with. Your taste buds and your gut will thank you.

Speaking of switching things up, the body also needs time to rest, even rest from eating. Most of us have been conditioned to view hunger as something to be avoided at all costs, and so we try to make sure that we get three full meals every day, as well as some snacks—often sacrificing nutrition on the altar of regular eating. But occasionally going a bit hungry is not bad for you; it is quite the opposite. Over the ages, humans have thrived on cycles of feast and famine. Throughout our years of hunting and gathering, we learned to eat, and then to fast for short periods while searching for more food. In recent years, more and more research has shown that alternating between regular eating and intermittent fasting is actually very good for the body, particularly for insulin and blood sugar regulation. Keeping things varied—skipping the odd breakfast, experimenting with brief fasts, and varying between high-fat and medium-fat diets—keeps the metabolism alert, and allows the body to regularly switch to fat-burning mode. This approach is called "metabolic switching," and it has been shown to contribute to mental clarity and improved cell healing (Pelz, 2022).

Intermittent fasting has become increasingly popular, and with all good reasons, but don't jump blindly into this approach if you have never heard of it before. Different bodies need different approaches, with male bodies generally faring better with a regular intermittent fasting routine, while women need more variation. Women, especially while still premenopausal, require different amounts of carbs at different times of the month, and should not fast for long when their progesterone levels are heightened. Do your research—Dr. Mindy Pelz's book, *Fast Like a Girl* (2022), can serve as a good starting point of research for women. You don't have to fast to be healthy, although it could be a wonderful addition to your life (if fasting speaks to you). Whatever you choose, however, I encourage you to rethink your relationship with hunger. Most of us don't just eat when we are hungry; we also eat when we are bored, scared, sad, or simply because it feels like a social thing to do. Becoming more conscious of your habits around food, or of the kinds of foods you grab when experiencing uncomfortable emotions, can be a huge step in the direction towards more healthy living.

Superfoods for Vitality and Wellness

You have probably heard of superfoods before—every few months, a new food makes it onto the cover of every wellness magazine, being touted as "the new best," the most nutritious food ever. Although mostly these reports are sensationalized, there is usually some truth in these reports. Some foods simply contain more nutrients than others, and massively benefit a host of organs and boost the immune system. Some of these foods have already popped up throughout this book: Turmeric and garlic, among others, feature strongly in almost any discussion of whole-body health. They are just good for you, almost regardless of your unique bodily needs, age, and situation. There are various other superfoods, too, some quite obscure, but commonly found, and all are tremendously good for you. Adding superfoods to your diet is a practical way of enriching your diet, and to experiment with flavors in the certainty that everything you are eating is benefiting your body. Here is a list of some superfoods (there are more out there, so make sure to do some additional research):

- **Blueberries:** Bursting with antioxidants, blueberries are renowned for their ability to combat oxidative stress and inflammation. These flavorful delights are rich in vitamins C and K, fiber, and manganese. Buy them in bulk when they are in season—blueberries freeze well, and defrost easily, so they can be enjoyed year-long in smoothies, oatmeal, or as a delicious snack.

- **Chia Seeds:** These tiny seeds are a treasure trove of omega-3 fatty acids, fiber, and antioxidants. They promote heart health, aid digestion, and provide a feeling of satiety, thus helping to prevent overeating.

Soak them for a while before eating—as else they might expand uncomfortably in your belly—then eat them by sprinkling on yogurt, blending into smoothies, or just as a nutritious chia pudding. They can also be used as sauce thickeners.

- **Quinoa:** This grain is considered a complete protein, which means that it contains all nine amino acids essential to the body. Quinoa is also high in fiber, iron, magnesium, and B vitamins. Use it as a base for salads, stir-fries, or as a nutritious alternative to rice or couscous.

- **Avocado:** This creamy fruit is rich in heart-healthy fats, fiber, and vitamins K, C, and E. Avocados offer a delicious and nutritious addition to salads, sandwiches, or as the star ingredient in guacamole. Eat them in season, which is when they taste best and leave a smaller carbon footprint, since importing these fruits can have quite an environmental impact otherwise.

- **Kale:** With its robust nutrient profile, kale is a nutritional powerhouse. It is packed with vitamins A, C, and K, as well as minerals like calcium and iron. Enjoy kale in salads, sautés, or as crispy kale chips. If you struggle to enjoy the taste of kale, try salting the fresh leaves and leaving them to sweat for a short while before adding them to the rest of your meal.

- **Cacao:** Raw cacao is a true superfood, packed with antioxidants, flavonoids, and magnesium. It can enhance mood, promote cardiovascular health, and provide a natural energy boost. Incorporate cacao nibs or unsweetened cocoa powder into smoothies, desserts, or homemade energy balls. Dark chocolate, as long as it is not too sweetened, is also a wonderful way of consuming cacao.

- **Broccoli:** This humble cruciferous vegetable is a nutritional powerhouse, brimming with vitamins C and K, fiber, and various antioxidants. Broccoli supports detoxification, immune function, and offers anti-inflammatory benefits. Enjoy it steamed, roasted, or sautéed as a tasty side dish or salad ingredient.

- **Almonds:** These crunchy nuts are rich in healthy fats, protein, fiber, vitamin E, and minerals like magnesium and calcium. Almonds can support heart health, satiety, and provide a satisfying snack option. Soak them overnight, then roast them or eat them raw as a standalone snack, sprinkle them over salads, or use them as a base for homemade nut butter.

- **Salmon:** As an oily fish, salmon provides a rich source of omega-3 fatty acids which supports heart health and brain function. It is also a great source of high-quality protein, vitamins B and D. Make sure you buy your salmon wild-caught, and also in the right season, since overfishing and unethical agricultural practices strongly affect the fishing industry. Other oily fish, such as trout and mackerel, also provide good alternatives. Grill, bake, or pan-sear salmon for a delectable and nutritious meal.

- **Greek Yogurt:** If you eat dairy, then yogurt should be one of your first nutritional ports of call. This versatile food is not only a great source of protein, but also contains probiotics that support gut health. Greek yogurt is rich in calcium, vitamin B12, and iodine. Enjoy it with fresh fruits, use it as a base for smoothies, or include it in savory sauces and dressings. I personally like using yogurt as a replacement for cream or milk, for everything from scrambled eggs to muesli.

- **Acai Berries:** These small, dark purple berries hail from the Amazon rainforest and are packed with antioxidants. Acai berries support heart health, promote healthy skin, and may have anti-inflammatory effects. Enjoy them in smoothie bowls, mixed into yogurt, or as a frozen treat.

- **Pomegranate:** Vibrant red and delicious, pomegranates are also a true antioxidant powerhouse. They are rich in polyphenols, which have been linked to heart health and help reduce inflammation. Pomegranates also provide vitamins C and K, as well as fiber. Buy them in season and enjoy them as a refreshing snack, add them to salads, or use the juice in smoothies and dressings.

Harnessing the Power of Herbs and Spices: A Flavorful Path to Health

Herbs and spices do more than just add depth and flavor to our dishes. They also possess remarkable health benefits that have been cherished and utilized for centuries. Most of them are rich in vitamins, minerals, and essential oils, all of which contributes to their unique health-promoting properties. Incorporating them into your cooking is an effective way of adding to the variety of your diet, while exploring different flavor profiles and possibilities. They can also be added to teas and infusions—in fact, that's one of my favorite ways of consuming various spices every day. When making a herb or spice infusion, a good rule of thumb is: The woodier the plant, the longer it should boil for its nutritional components to be effectively extracted. A fresh herb only needs to steep for a few minutes, while dried herbs should boil for a while, and spices such as cloves and ginger can be allowed to boil for hours, or until the water volume has been halved.

We have discussed various herbs and spices throughout this book. Oregano, rosemary, holy basil, fennel, and thyme have all featured as wonderful herbs to add to everything: from salads to teas, relishes or even stews. Spices such as allspice, turmeric, ginger, and cinnamon are also hugely beneficial. Apart from these and several others that have been already discussed, here are some more beneficial herbs and spices you could incorporate into your meals:

- **Dill:** Known for its delicate feathery leaves and distinct flavor, dill is related to fennel, but tastes rather different, making it a good substitute if you are not fond of the liquorice taste of fennel. It is a good source of vitamin A and C, and minerals like calcium and iron. Dill possesses antimicrobial properties and can aid digestion, alleviate menstrual discomfort, and support bone health. It pairs wonderfully with fish, roasted vegetables, and dressings.

- **Caraway Seeds:** These small aromatic seeds come from the caraway plant and have a warm, slightly sweet taste. Caraway seeds are rich in antioxidants, fiber, and essential oils. They are known to aid digestion, relieve bloating and gas, and also have antimicrobial and anti-inflammatory effects. Caraway seeds are commonly used in bread, sauerkraut, and traditional dishes like rye bread and goulash. I also like to sprinkle them into rice or quinoa before cooking it, for a sweetly tangy aroma.

- **Cilantro:** This is a versatile herb widely used in various cuisines, and can easily be grown on your windowsill. It offers a fresh, citrusy flavor and is a good source of vitamin K, vitamin C, and antioxidants. Also known as coriander, it helps support digestion, lower cholesterol levels, and bears antimicrobial properties. It can be used as a garnish, added to salsas, curries, and salads, or infused into teas.

- **Coriander Seeds:** Derived from the same plant as cilantro, coriander seeds have a warm, earthy flavor. These seeds are rich in antioxidants and have been traditionally used to promote easier digestion, reduce inflammation, and support blood sugar control. They can be used in spice blends, added to soups and stews, or crushed and sprinkled over roasted vegetables.

- **Mustard Seeds:** Mustard seeds come in various colors, including yellow, brown, and black, all of which have a distinctive, pungent flavor. Mustard seeds are a good source of omega-3 fatty acids, antioxidants, and minerals like selenium and magnesium. They are believed to have antimicrobial and anti-inflammatory properties, aid digestion, and promote heart health. Mustard seeds can be used in dressings, marinades, pickles, or grounded into mustard paste.

- **Star Anise:** This star-shaped spice has a unique sweet and licorice-like flavor. It contains essential oils, antioxidants, and compounds with potential antimicrobial and anti-inflammatory properties. Star anise is commonly used in Asian cuisine, especially in soups, broths, and spice blends like Chinese Five Spice. It adds depth to both savory and sweet dishes. It is also one of my favorite ingredients for homemade chai tea, along with ginger and cloves.

- **Cloves:** Cloves are known for their warm, aromatic flavor and potent medicinal properties. They contain eugenol, a compound with antioxidant and anti-inflammatory effects. Cloves aid digestion, alleviate toothaches, kill internal parasites and provide respiratory support. They are commonly used in spice blends, stews, desserts, and mulled drinks.

- **Parsley:** Often used as a garnish, parsley is a versatile herb with a fresh, vibrant flavor. It is an excellent source of vitamin K and C and antioxidants. Parsley may support heart health, help detoxify the body, and have anti-inflammatory effects. It can be added to salads, soups, sauces, and pesto, or simply picked from your garden and eaten immediately— they freshen both the breath and the mind.

- **Cayenne Pepper:** This fiery spice derived from chili peppers is famous for its heat and vibrant red color. Cayenne pepper contains a compound known for its metabolism-boosting properties, and it aids digestion, promotes cardiovascular health, and provides pain relief. Cayenne pepper can be added to spice up various dishes, sauces, and marinades—in fact, it can be sprinkled over everything, from scrambled eggs to your regular coffee.

Conclusion

As we reach the end of this transformative journey toward wellness, it is important to reflect over the principles we have explored together. Throughout this book, we have embraced the power of nature, the wisdom of ancient healing practices, and the innate connection between mind, body, and spirit. We have discovered that true wellbeing lies in our ability to take charge of our own health, and nurture our bodies with the gifts that nature provides.

In a world filled with distractions and fragmented approaches to wellness, it is easy to feel overwhelmed and disconnected. But each of us holds the key to our own wellbeing, and the choices we make each day have a profound impact on our health. In the pages of this book, we have delved into nutritional practices backed both by science and folk medicine, and saw how much healing can be obtained through simple actions such as movement, diverse eating, and embracing the power of herbs and spices. We have also explored the remarkable potential of natural resources: from the healing properties of plants to the transformative power of mindfulness and deep breathing.

As we conclude this journey now, I invite you to carry forward the lessons and practices you have discovered today. Take responsibility for your own wellbeing, recognizing that you have the power to make positive changes in your life (and others). Listen to the whispers of your body, trust your intuition, and honor your unique needs. Embrace the interconnectedness of your being and the interconnectedness of all beings on this planet.

Remember, holistic wellness is not a destination, but an ongoing, lifelong journey. It requires a commitment to self-care, self-discovery, and self-love. Nurture your body, mind, and spirit with the abundance of resources that nature provides. Seek balance, discover joy, and cultivate gratitude for the miracles of life. You are the author of your own wellbeing, and the choices you make today will shape your health tomorrow. Embrace this responsibility with courage and grace, and let your journey toward vibrant wellbeing continue to unfold.

References

7 Signs of a Healthy Heart. (2018, February 20). *7 signs of a healthy heart.* Integra Urgent Care. https://integrauc.com/blog/7-signs-healthy-heart/

Allen, S. (2018). *The science of gratitude.* Greater Good Science Center. https://ggsc.berkeley.edu/images/uploads/GGSC-JTF_White_Paper-Gratitude-FINAL.pdf

Buettner, D. (2010). *The blue zones: Lessons for living longer from the people who've lived the longest.* National Geographic Society.

Butter vs. Margarine. (2020, January 29). *Butter vs. margarine.* Harvard Health. https://www.health.harvard.edu/staying-healthy/butter-vs-margarine

Bush, Z. (2020, January 12). *What exactly is the skin's microbiome?* HAPPI. https://www.happi.com/contents/view_experts-opinion/2020-12-01/what-exactly-is-the-skins-microbiome/

Cummings, G. (2017, August 31). *10 common digestive herbs and how they benefit your health.* Evening Standard. Www.standard.co.uk.https://www.standard.co.uk/reveller/foodanddrink/10-common-digestive-herbs-and-how-they-benefit-your-health-a3624266.html

Delagran, L. (2011). *How does nature impact our wellbeing? Taking Charge of Your Health & Wellbeing.* https://www.takingcharge.csh.umn.edu/how-does-nature-impact-our-wellbeing

Enders, J. (2015). *Gut: The inside story of our body's most underrated organ.* Greystone Books.

Essential Oils for Your Hair. (2022, December 6). *Essential oils for your hair.* WebMD. https://www.webmd.com/beauty/natural-oils

Frankl, V. E. (2006). *Man's search for meaning.* Beacon Press. (Original work published 1946).

Gladstar, R. (2008). *Rosemary Gladstar's herbal recipes for vibrant health: 175 teas, tonics, oils, salves, tinctures, and other natural remedies for the entire family.* Storey Pub.

Hand, E. (2016, July 16). *Can hair change from straight to curly?* Science World. https://www.scienceworld.ca/stories/can-hair-change-straight-curly/

Hollister, S. (2017). *Natural hair care.* Createspace Independent Publishing Platform.

Hoss, E. (2021, April 14). *Male pattern baldness.* Penn Medicine. https://www.pennmedicine.org/for-patients-and-visitors/patient-information/conditions-treated-a-to-z/male-pattern-baldness

Is Broken Heart Syndrome Real? (2022, April 4). *Is broken heart syndrome real?* American Heart Association. https://www.heart.org/en/health-topics/cardiomyopathy/what-is-cardiomyopathy-in-adults/is-broken-heart-syndrome-real

Jones, T. (2023, February 14). *The 12 best foods for healthy skin.* Healthline. https://www.healthline.com/nutrition/12-foods-for-healthy-skin

Kaplan, S. (1995). The restorative benefits of nature: Toward an integrative framework. *Journal of Environmental Psychology, 15*(3), 169–182. https://doi.org/10.1016/0272-4944(95)90001-2

Mergenthaler, P., Lindauer, U., Dienel, G. A., & Meisel, A. (2013). Sugar for the brain: the role of glucose in physiological and pathological brain function. *Trends in Neurosciences, 36*(10), 587–597. https://doi.org/10.1016/j.tins.2013.07.001

Pelz, M. (2022). *Fast like a girl.* Hay House, Inc.

Reynolds, S. (2021, March 9). *Cells that maintain and repair the liver identified.* National Institutes of Health (NIH). https://www.nih.gov/news-events/nih-research-matters/cells-maintain-repair-liver-identified

Rivas, G. (2022, November 7). *Is your scalp oily, dry, or balanced? Here's how to know—and the best way to take care of your scalp type.* Real Simple. https://www.realsimple.com/beauty-fashion/hair/hair-care/scalp-types

Sissons, B. (2023, May 17). *The 9 best herbs for joint pain.* Medical News Today. https://www.medicalnewstoday.com/articles/

The Focus is on Foot Health with Pivotal Motion Physiotherapy. (2018, July 01). *The focus is on foot health with pivotal motion physiotherapy.* Pivotal

Motion. https://pivotalmotion.physio/the-focus-is-on-foot-health-with-pivotal-motion-physiotherapy/

Thye, A. Y.-K., Bah, Y.-R., Law, J. W.-F., Tan, L. T.-H., He, Y.-W., Wong, S.-H., Thurairajasingam, S., Chan, K.-G., Lee, L.-H., & Letchumanan, V. (2022). Gut–Skin axis: Unravelling the connection between the gut microbiome and psoriasis. *Biomedicines, 10*(5), 1037. https://doi.org/10.3390/biomedicines10051037

van der Kolk, B. (2014). *The body keeps the score: Mind, brain and body in the transformation of trauma*. Penguin Books.

Vaughn, A. R., Branum, A., & Sivamani, R. K. (2016). Effects of turmeric (Curcuma longa) on skin health: A systematic review of the clinical evidence. *Phytotherapy Research, 30*(8), 1243–1264. https://doi.org/10.1002/ptr.5640

Water Science School. (2019, May 22). *The water in you: Water and the human body*. U.S. Geological Survey. https://www.usgs.gov/special-topics/water-science-school/science/water-you-water-and-human-body

Watson, K. (2019, October 23). *Everything You Need to Know About Flavonoids*. Healthline. https://www.healthline.com/health/what-are-flavonoids-everything-you-need-to-know

Wells, D., & Collins, D. (2022, April 6). *How to fix neck pain: Stiff neck causes, treatment, and prevention*. Healthline. https://www.healthline.com/health/how-to-get-rid-of-a-stiff-neck#when-to-see-a-doctor

What's in a Bar of Soap? (2016, April 25). *What's in a bar of soap?* Bare-Soaps. https://www.bare-soaps.com/blogs/your-impact/116431557-what-s-in-a-bar-of-soap

Why do we hold so much tension in our neck and shoulders? (n.d.). *Why do we hold so much tension in our neck and shoulders?* Intulo Health. http://www.intulohealth.com/intulo-health-blog-articles/remedial-massage-and-body-mot-articles/62-tension-in-our-neck-and-shoulders

Williams, J. (2023, April 12). *Eat your way to fabulous skin*. BBC Good Food. https://www.bbcgoodfood.com/howto/guide/eat-your-way-fabulous-skin

Winston, D., & Maimes, S. (2019). *Adaptogens: herbs for strength, stamina, and stress relief*. Healing Arts Press.

Yu, S. H., & Park, S. D. (2015). The effects of a neck musculoskeletal intervention on neck pain levels and depression in post-traumatic stress disorder patients. *Journal of Physical Therapy Science, 27*(6), 1975–1978. https://doi.org/10.1589/jpts.27.1975

Printed in Great Britain
by Amazon

31416165R00076